Molecular Mechanisms of COPD-Associated Osteoporosis

S.Krishna

Title: **Molecular Mechanisms of COPD-Associated Osteoporosis**

Author's: **S.Krishn**

This book was printed and published by [Publisher's: S.**Krishn**] in [2023]

ISBN: 9781805250661

CONTENTS

LIST OF TABLES

LIST OF FIGURES

ABBREVIATIONS

AP-1	activating protein 1
AR	androgen receptor
B-fgf	basic fibroblast growth factor
BSA	bovine serum albumin
CXCR4	Chemokine receptor type 4
cAMP	Cyclic Adenosine Monophosphate
COPD	Chronic obstructive pulmonary disease
DMEM	Dulbecco's modified Eagle's medium
ECM	extracellular matrix
EGF	epidermal growth factor
EGFR	epidermal growth factor receptor
ERKs	extracellular signal-regulated kinases
FAC	focal adhesion complex
FAK	focal adhesion kinase
FBS	Fetal bovine serum
Fra - 1	Fos-related antigen 1
GAP	GTPase-activating protein
GDI	GDP dissociation inhibitor
GSH	reduced glutathione
ICAM	intercellular adhesion molecule
IKK	IκB kinase
IKB	NF-κB inhibitory protein
IL	interleukin
JNK	c-Jun N-terminal kinase
MAPK	mitogen activated protein kinase
MAPKK	mitogen activated protein kinase kinase
MAPKKK	mitogen activated protein kinase kinase kinase
MTT	4,5-Dimethylthiazol-2-yl)-2,5-Diphenyltetrazolium Bromide
MMP	matrix metalloproteinase

NF-κB	nuclear factor kappaB
PAK	p21-activated kinase
PBMCs	Peripheral blood mononuclear cell
PDGF	Platelet-derived growth factor
PI3K	Phosphatidylinositol 3-kinase
PIP2	phosphatidylinositol 4,5-bisphosphate
PIP3	phosphatidylinositol (3,4,5)-triphosphate
PKA	protein kinase A
PKC	protein kinase C
PLCβ	Phospholipase C-β
PLCγ-1	Phospholipase C-γ
RT-PCR	Reverse transcription polymerase chain reaction
SDS-PAGE	Sodium Dodecyl Sulfate Polyacrylamide Gel Electrophoresis.
TGF-β1	transforming growth factor beta1
TIMP	tissue inhibitors of MMPs
TNF-α	tumor necrosis factor alpha
CTR	CTR - Calcitonin receptor
RANKL	Receptor Activator for Nuclear Factor (NF)- κB Ligand
TRAP	Tartrate-resistant acid phosphatase
MBC	Metastatic breast cancer
MDR	Multi drug resistance
mRNA	Messenger Ribonucleic Acid
TRAP	Tartrate-resistant acid phosphatase
ERα	Estrogen receptor alpha
ERβ	Estrogen receptor beta
PBMCs	Peripheral blood mononuclear cells
WHO	World Health Organisation.
DALYS	Disability Adjusted Life Years.
GBD	Global Burden of Diesease
PTH	Para Thyroid Hormone
M-CSF	Macrrophage Colony Stimulating Factor
MSC	Mesenchymal Stem Cells

OPG	OsteoProtegerin.
FADD	Fas Associated Death Domain Protein
Pro – CATK	Pro Cathepsin K
TRAF	TNF Receptor Associated Factor
FEV1	Forced Expired Volume in 1 second.
FVC	Forced Vital Capacity.
TBS	Tris Buffered Saline.
TBST	Tris Buffered Saline + Tween 20.
ERK	Extra Cellular Signal – Regulated Kinase.
JNK	C-Jun N-Terminal Kinase.
Bcl – 2	B-Cell Lymphoma – 2
PTK	Protein Tyrosine Kinase.
APS	Ammonium per sulphate

INTRODUCTION

Chronic Obstructive Pulmonary Disease (COPD)

COPD is striking by hampering the normal breathing due to chronic obstruction of airflow to the lungs. Alternatively, COPD comprises the distinct pathological condition of both chronic bronchitis and emphysema. Permanent complications arise and persist in COPD and worsening over time, making it virtually non curable. COPD is caused by the long term exposure to lung irritants such as cigarette, pipe, cigar and other types of tobacco smoke, second hand smoke, chemical fumes or fumes from burning fuel for cooking, air pollution and dust from the environment or workplace, and a genetic condition resulting in alpha-antitrypsin deficiency.

Prevalence of COPD

COPD is a leading cause of morbidity and mortality worldwide, especially among smokers over 40 years of age and individuals exposed to biomass smoke (Rabe *et al.,* 2007). The World Health Organization estimates that COPD will be the third most common worldwide cause of death and disability by 2030, from its current fifth ranking (WHO, 2014). Despite worldwide medical research, health care efforts, and health care costs, COPD statistics reveal a continuing upward trend in mortality, in contrast with other major causes of death like cancer and cardiovascular disease (WHO, 2014). The global prevalence of COPD was measured to be approximately 9-10 percent in adults aged $\geq$40 years. It is reported as 6th and 5th leading cause of death in 1990 and 2002 respectively and leading to become the 3rd by the year 2020. It is also ranked 12th for cause of disability-adjusted life years (DALYS, defines as the number of years lost due to ill-health, disability or early death) in 1990 and is projected to become the 5th by 2020. COPD is ranked 5th with DALYS in the Netherlands and is the 4th leading cause of death in the United States. More than 30% rise in total deaths from COPD is expected in the next 10 years. Burden of Obstructive Lung Disease (BOLD) study from 12 sites engaging 9425 subjects to determine the international variation in the prevalence of COPD by Buist *et al.*, estimated that the overall prevalence of GOLD stage II or higher COPD was 10.1 per cent with 11.8 per cent for men and 8.5 per cent for women (Buist *et al.*, 2007). Halbert *et al.*, reviewed population-based prevalence estimates and published during the period (1990-2004) and found that South-east Asia is having a high prevalence (11.4%) for COPD and noted a few other geographical zones which includes America (4.6%), Europe (28%), and pacific zones (4%) in his study .

Age and smoking are the major risk factors for COPD and a number of other illnesses, often leading to COPD patients demonstrating multiple coexisting morbidities (Chatila *et al.*, 2008; Tsiligianni *et al.*, 2013). Older people are more susceptible to COPD and are highly prevalent among those aged more than 75 yr. A study by Parasuramalu *et al.*, on the prevalence of COPD revealed that the prevalence was increasing proportionally with age, i.e., 2.5%, 3.85%, 6.72% and 9.52% prevalence in 35-44 years, 45-54 years, 55-64 years and 65-74 years respectively (Parasuramalu *et al.*, 2014).

Indian prevalence of COPD

COPD and Asthma are the most common diseases in India. COPD is one of the leading non-communicable causes of death globally, as well as in India (GBD 2015; GBD 2017; ICMR 2017). India has a population of 1.3 billion people living in 29 states and seven union territories, many of which have populations as large as some countries, and which often vary widely in terms of ecology, economy, and demography, all of which affect respiratory health(Government of India, 2017). The Sustainable Development Goals aim to reduce premature mortality from noncommunicable diseases by one third by 2030 through prevention and treatment (United nations, 2018). The National Health Policy of India 2017 recommends that premature mortality from non-communicable diseases, including chronic respiratory diseases, should be reduced by 25% by 2025 (Ministry of Health and Family Welfare, Government of India, 2017). Health is a state subject in the Indian federal structure, with most health expenditure coming from state budgets (Ministry of Health and

Family Welfare, 2018). In 2017, the India State-Level Disease Burden Initiative reported a varied epidemiological transition occurring among the states of India from 1990 to 2016 as part of the Global Burden of Diseases, Injuries, and Risk Factors Study (GBD) 2016.(2,3)

India over the past quarter century, prevalence has increased leading to its ranking now, as the second leading individual cause of Disease Burden in India. With 18% of the global population, India has a disproportionately high 32% of the global disability adjusted life years (DALYS) from chronic respiratory diseases. In 2016, the prevalence of COPD in India was 4.2% and the prevalence of asthma 2.9%. India has a prevalence of COPD that is higher than the global average, as well as more DALYS per person with COPD or asthma than the global average. Most states in India had higher rates of DALYS from COPD and asthma compared with locations elsewhere in the world at similar levels of SDI. However, there were substantial variations between the states. The case-fatality rates for COPD and asthma decreased across all ETL state groups from 1990 to 2016, but these rates were twice as high in the less developed low ETL state group than in the high ETL state group in 2016. The DALY rate due to COPD varied four fold between the states, and that of asthma three fold. Rajasthan and Uttar Pradesh in north India, both of which are in the low ETL state group, had the highest DALY rates of COPD and asthma in 2016. From 1990 to 2016, the crude prevalence of COPD in India increased by 29% and that of asthma by 9%. However, age-standardized prevalence declined by 5% for COPD and 4% for asthma. This finding suggests that the overall increases in prevalence are mainly due to ageing of the population in India. Understanding changes in the risk factors for COPD, which makes up three-quarters of the chronic respiratory disease burden in India, would be instructive for placing the changes in prevalence in perspective. The dominant risk factor for COPD in India in 2016 was air pollution, which contributed more than half the DALYS due to COPD, followed by smoking, which contributed a quarter of the COPD DALYs. As described previously by the India State-Level Disease Burden Initiative, ambient air pollution exposure has increased in most parts of India since 1990, whereas exposure to household air pollution has decreased because of a reduction in the use of solid fuels, although it is still quite high (GBD, 2017; ICMR, 2017).

Despite decline in basic and age-standardized DALYS rates of COPD and asthma, suggesting improvements in health care, India still has substantially higher DALYS per person with COPD and asthma than the global average. This high rate of health loss from COPD is due to issues related to its relatively late diagnosis and management, even with the improvements in health care over time in India. Evidence suggests that COPD is underdiagnosed in India, partly because diagnosis is mostly based on symptoms rather than spirometry and also because symptomatic people are often late in seeking care because of insufficient awareness of the disease (Salvi *et al.*, 2012; Gupta *et al.*, 2013). The prescription of inhalation devices, which is often needed to manage the late stages of COPD, is often perceived as a stigma in rural areas (Gupta *et al.*, 2013). Most symptomatic individuals tend to seek treatment from the non-formal health practitioners of alternative medicines and faith healing, who often prescribe harmful and toxic agents. Women at the early stages of the disease are less symptomatic than men, which, combined with their less common health seeking behavior, poses additional challenges to COPD diagnosis (Kalagouda *et al.*, 2016).

Table 1.1: Prevalence studies on COPD among various regional populations in India are clustered (Vijayan and Nice 2012)

Area	Prevalence in Men (%)	Prevalence in Women (%)
Rural Delhi	3.36	2,54
Patna	2.12	1.33
New Delhi	8.1	4.6
Madras	1.9	1.2
North Arcot District,Tamilnadu	4.08	2.55

Jindal *et al.*, reported that the prevalence of COPD in rural and urban areas of north India was 6.2 % in men and 3.9 % in women and 4.2 % in men and 1.6 % in women respectively (Jindal *et al.*, 1993). INSEARCH study by Jindal *et al* found the overall prevalence of chronic bronchitis in Indian cities is 3.49% in adults aged ≥35 years (Jindal *et al.*, 2012).

Table 1.2: Results from INSEARCH study on the prevalence of chronic Bronchitis in various cities (Jindal *et al.*, 2012).

Cities	Prevalence (%)
Ahmedabad	4.8
Berhampur	1.9
Bikaner	5.7
Chennai	2.7
Guwahati	2.1
Kolkata	3.7
Mumbai	1.1
Mysore	2.1
Nagpur	1.2
Secundrabad	1.6
Shimla	1.7

Burden on health care costs

COPD remains a major health issue with a significant economic impact (Valente *etal.*, 2010). The prevalence of COPD is rising in developing and developed countries, resulting in increased direct and indirect costs of COPD to health care systems worldwide. In the USA, direct costs have escalated from 18 billion dollars in

2002 to 29.5 billion in 2010, the largest part consisting of hospital expenses, whereas indirect costs accounted for 27% - 61% of total costs, with the higher estimates produced by studies of working age populations (Pasquale *et al.*, 2010;

Ornek *et al.*, 2012; Patel *et al.*, 2014). The total annual direct costs of COPD expenditure are directly associated with the number of comorbidities, not the severity of airflow obstruction or health-related quality of life indices (Halpin *et al.*, 2006; Mapel *et al.*, 2000). Comorbidities, after age and chronic symptoms, are the factors most predictive of future health care costs (Simon *et al.*, 2011). COPD patients with comorbidities have increased risk and significantly higher mean costs for hospital admissions (Mannino *et al.*, 2006).

Complications of COPD

COPD is an inflammatory disorder characterized by persistent and progressive airflow which is attributable not only to the lung disease, but also to systemic complications which include osteoporosis, loss of skeletal muscle mass and function, systemic inflammation, catabolic intermediary metabolism, impaired glucose tolerance, and an increased risk of cardiovascular disease, all of which cause considerable morbidity and mortality (Agusti *et al.*, 2008; Rabe *et al.*, 2007; Almagro *et al.*, 2014; Negewo *et al.*, 2015).

Osteoporosis

Osteoporosis, a condition characterized by low bone mass and bone micro architectural deterioration which predisposes to fragility fracture, is one of the most important systemic complications of COPD and is associated with poor health status and prognosis (Nussbaumer *et al.*, 2011). The incidence of osteoporosis among COPD patients is significantly higher than in the general population and this association is not limited to those with severe COPD (Kjensli *et al.*, 2007; Vrieze *et al.*, 2007). The mechanisms underlying bone loss in COPD are multifactorial, and systemic inflammation is believed to play a central role, but it remains unclear how systemic inflammation interacts with bone metabolism, and what are the culprit cells and molecules in this complex process (Biskobing *et al.,* 2002; Divo *et al.,* 2015; Barnes *et al.,* 2009; Sinden *et al.,* 2010). However, the pathophysiology appears to be at least partially independent of exposure to glucocorticoids. For example, Bolton *et al.,* reported a high prevalence of osteoporosis in patients with COPD who were not receiving long-term oral corticosteroid therapy (Bolton *et al.,* 2009).

In a study performed by Duckers *et al.,* over 80% of the male COPD patients with predominantly mild to moderate airflow obstruction (GOLD I and II) had osteopenia or osteoporosis (Duckers *et al.,* 2011). Likewise, Sin *et al.,* found that, in non-Hispanic Caucasians, airflow obstruction was associated with decreased bone mineral density. Thirty-three percent of female patients with severe COPD suffered from osteoporosis, while almost all women with relatively mild airway obstruction suffered from osteopenia (Sin *et al.,* 2003). Clinical sequel of osteoporosis, including thoracic compression fractures and kyphosis, can further reduce vital capacity, thereby further compromising respiratory status in patients with COPD (Leech *et al.,* 1990). WHO characterized osteoporosis based on the bone mass density (BMD), if the value is >2.5 standard deviations (SD) below the young adult mean. If BMD is between 1 and 2.5 SDs below the mean for young adults, a pre- clinical condition of osteoporosis called osteopenia is defined.

Types of osteoporosis

Primary osteoporosis include bone loss due to age-related loss of gonadal function in women and the aging process in men, and bone loss due to other chronic diseases and the effect of medications leads to secondary osteoporosis.

Primary osteoporosis

Primary osteoporosis is classified into postmenopausal osteoporosis and senile osteoporosis.

Postmenopausal osteoporosis

Postmenopausal osteoporosis is caused by the estrogen deficiency making the skeleton more receptive to parathyroid hormone (PTH) and calcium resorption is increased as a result which in turn decreases the secretion of PTH, 1,25-dihydroxyvitamin D production, and calcium absorption leading to the trabecular bone loss causing vertebral crush and colles' fractures (Riggs and Melton 1986). Further, estrogen indirectly influences the bone metabolism through cytokines and local growth factors. Osteoclast apoptosis may increase in the estrogen-wealth condition through the secretion of the transforming growth factor (TGF)-beta. A study on ovariectomized mice indicates an increase in the levels of IL-6 and GM-CFU implying, inhibition of IL-6 by the estrogen. As the estrogen depletes, T-cell secrets IL-1, IL-6 and TNF-alpha, thereby encouraging the recruitment, differentiation and prolonged survival of osteoclasts, exhibiting its contribution to osteoporosis (Jilka *et al.*, 1992), additionally estrogen deficiency causes premature apoptosis of osteoblast and inhibition of osteoblast differentiation through the production of cytokines such as IL-17 by T-cells. Significant depletion in estrogen production in women results in 50% trabecular bone and 35% cortical bone loss throughout their lifetime, whereas men experience 25% of both types of bone (Riggs and Melton 1986).

Senile osteoporosis

With senile osteoporosis, the bone loss is associated with the decrease in the bone formation caused by a drop in osteoblast supply compared to the demand which is determined by the number of new cycles of remodelling are initiated. After 30 years, bone resorption exceeds bone formation that leads to senile osteoporosis. In addition, kidney failed to produce sufficient 1,25 (OH) 2D3 causing vitamin D deficiency leading to the cascade of decreased calcium absorption, increased PTH level, increased bone resorption leading to cortical and trabecular bone loss (Iqbal 2000).

Risk factors for primary osteoporosis

Lifestyle causes like sedentary lifestyle, excessive alcohol consumption, tobacco use, low calcium intake, anorexia, and physical inactivity lead to lower bone density. People with impaired neuromuscular function are with the risk for developing fragility fractures. Amenorrhea, Gastrointestinal surgery, lower sex hormones, increased thyroid hormone levels, low body weight and weight loss are associated with greater bone loss and increased risk of fracture. Weight in infancy is found to be a determinant of bone mass in adulthood. Men and women either middle-aged or older with annual height loss >0.5 cm are at increased risk of fractures of any kind especially hip fracture.

Secondary osteoporosis

Secondary osteoporosis results as an extended complication of many chronic diseases and caused by the usage of drugs prescribed for its treatment that interfere with the attainment of peak bone mass and increase the bone loss.

Medical condition that lead to secondary osteoporosis

Serious kidney failure, Cushing's disease (a tumor of the pituitary gland, responsible for secreting some of the body's hormones), Liver impairment, Anorexia nervosa and bulimia, Rheumatoid arthritis, Malabsorption syndromes such as Crohn's disease, ulcerative colitis and Celiac disease, Chronic obstructive pulmonary disease (a condition affecting the airways), Scurvy, Hyperparathyroidism, Hyperthyroidism, Diabetes, Hypercortisolism, Thalassemia: a hereditary form of anemia, Multiple myeloma: multiple tumors within the bone and bone marrow, Leukemia, Neurological disorders such as cerebral palsy, Multiple sclerosis, Parkinson's disease, Neuropathy and Metastatic bone diseases.

Medications that cause secondary osteoporosis

Synthetic Glucocorticoids (e.g. prednisone), breast Cancer Drugs, Prostate Cancer Drugs, "heartburn" Drugs, Depo-Provera, Excessive Thyroid Hormone Replacement, Anti-seizure and Mood-altering Drugs, Blood Pressure Medication, Diuretics, Lithium (used to treat many psychiatric disorders), Acetaminophen (e.g. Tylenol®) for a period of at least 3 years, Narcotic and opioid medications, Barbiturates, Aluminium-containing antacids, Thiazolidinedione such as rosiglitazone, Antirejection/immunosuppressive therapy, Heparin (blood thinner), Anxiolytics, Sedatives, Neuroleptics and Anti-depressants.

Global prevalence of osteoporosis

Nearly, 200 million women are affected by osteoporosis worldwide at the rate of one-tenth aged 60, one-fifth aged 70, two-fifth aged 80 and two-third aged 90 and an estimated 75 million people were from Europe, USA and Japan. The residual lifetime risk of experiencing an osteoporotic fracture in men over the age of 50 is 27% and from the age of 60 is 25%, and in women above the age of 60 is 44%. Every year osteoporosis accounts for above 8.9 million fractures, at the rate of 1 fracture per 3 seconds. Approximately, 9 million new osteoporotic fractures were recorded in the year 2000 which consists of 1.7 million fractures at forearm, 1.6 million fractures at the hip and 1.4 million were clinical vertebral fractures, about 51% of all these fractures are credited to Europe and America. The projected incidence of hip fracture by the year 2050 is a 240% increase in women and 310% in men, i.e., an estimated rise to 6.26 million fractures combined, by the year 2050 worldwide (Johnell and Kanis 2004).

Prevalence of osteoporosis in India

India hosts approximately 26 million osteoporosis patients by 2003 with an estimated increase to 36 million by 2013 (Indumati *et al.*, 2007). Indian women aged 30-60 years from low income groups have BMD (at all the skeletal sites) lower than the values reported from developed countries, with a high prevalence of osteopenia (52%) and osteoporosis (29%) (Shatrugna *et al.*, 2005).

The hip fracture incidence were 159 and 105 per 100,000 per year in women and men, respectively, above the age of 50 years (Dhanwal *et al.*, 2013) and the prevalence of vertebral fractures were 17.9 % (males 18.8 %, females 17.1%) in a study subjects with a mean age of 64.9 (±.7) years (Marwaha *et al.*, 2012). A study on south Indian population found that the overall prevalence of osteoporosis at any one site was 20% and that of osteopenia was 58% (Shetty *et al.*, 2014).

COPD and OSTEOPOROSIS

COPD is one of the chronic diseases that facilitate the development of secondary osteoporosis. Prevalence of osteoporosis is 2 to 5 fold higher in COPD patients compared to normal patients (Ciric *et al.*, 2012) and the degree of the loss of BMD has been found to be proportionate to the COPD severity (Abu-Bakr *et al.*, 2014). COPD patients with low BMD have 3-fold increase in fracture risk(Abu- Bakr *et al.*, 2014) with 24%-63% prevalence for vertebral compression fractures, depending on the population studied (Lehouck *et al.*, 2011), which is more common than the lumbar fractures in all patients (Biskobing DM 2002).

Development of osteoporosis in COPD patients

Earlier, the prolonged use of corticosteroids, prescribed for treating COPD, is claimed for the development of osteoporosis with an increase in risk for non - vertebral fractures. Patients on long term corticosteroid therapy are at an increased risk of hip fractures by 2-fold and 2.6 fold in women and men respectively with the prevalence of 30-50%. Subsequently, it was found that the prevalence of osteoporosis is still high in the corticosteroid naive COPD patients, this entails the participation of more complex mechanism that drives the progression of secondary osteoporosis in COPD patients.

COPD patients are under a state of continuous systemic inflammation including a protein catabolic process involving increased production of catalytic enzymes (matrix metalloproteinases etc.), which together with the inflammatory cytokines like TNF-alpha, IL-1, and IL-6 causing bone resorption by inducing the expression of RANKL leading to osteoporosis (Sarkar *et al.*, 2015). Increased activity of alkaline phosphatase was found in the sera of COPD patients which may indicate the increased bone metabolism (Abu-Bakr *et al.*, 2014).

Pathogenesis of Osteoporosis in COPD

Bone is a dynamic tissue and in a continuous process of wear and tear. Modeling and remodeling has an important role to play in maintaining a healthy skeleton. Remodeling is the physiological process of new bone formation by the osteoblasts preceded by the osteoclasts-mediated bone resorption (Brandi *et al.*, 2009). Bone modeling, on the other hand, is characterized by the process of bone formation but not preceded by prior bone resorption. It is estimated that about 25% of trabecular bone and about 3% of cortical bone are replaced in adults every year (Lehouck *et al.*, 2011). Parathyroid hormone (PTH), vitamin D, and gonadal hormones are the key regulators of bone formation and resorption.

Osteoporosis develops because of an imbalance between bone formation and bone resorption, either excessive resorption or decreased formation. Osteoblasts, osteoclasts, and osteocytes interactions are important for the process of bone remodeling. Osteoclasts are multinucleate giant cells derived from blood monocytes/macrophage lineage. Osteo-clastogenesis is stimulated by the monocytes/macrophage colony-stimulating factor (M-CSF) and the receptor activator of nuclear factor-κ B (RANK)-ligand (RANKL) (Steiner *et al.*, 2011). Osteoclasts function as bone eaters by secreting a mixture of hydrogen and chloride ions and proteolytic enzymes. By secreting hydrogen ions, they make an acidic microenvironment, which is necessary for the activation of proteolytic enzymes that subsequently dissolve the bone collagen. Bone resorption helps in the clearance of micro damaged bone tissue and makes the foundation for the laying of new bones (Fig. 1).

Osteoblasts are derived from the mesenchymal stem cells (MSCs) and form new bones (Sims *et al.,* 2008). Osteocytes are the cells that initiate bone remodeling as these cells detect micro damages within the bone. Osteocytes after detecting the micro damages communicate with the osteoblasts and osteoclasts, which in turn initiate bone remodelling (Zuo *et al.,* 2012).

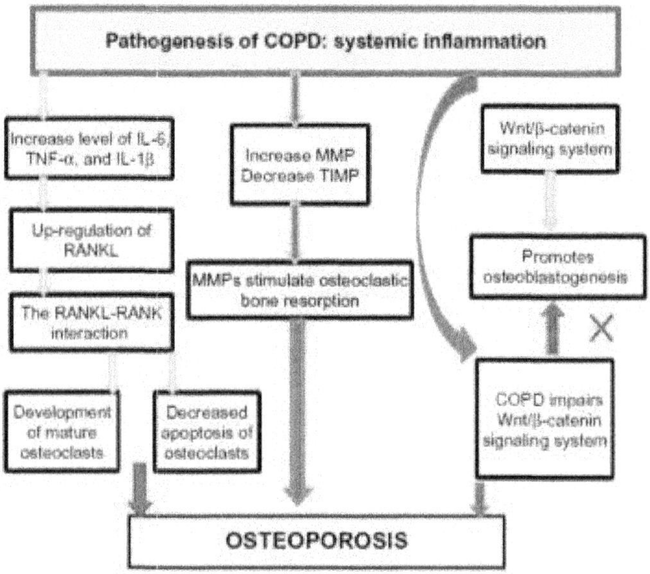

Figure 1. Pathogenesis of osteoporosis in COPD

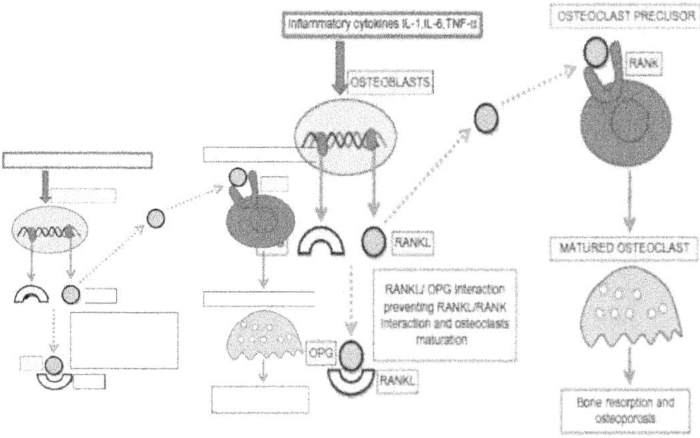

Figure 2. Relationship between RANK, RANKL and OPG

Osteoprotegerin (OPG)/RANK/RANKL Axis

OPG, RANK, and RANKL systems, also known as the OPG/ RANK/RANKL axis, play a critical role in the pathogenesis of osteoporosis. RANKL expressed on the surface of osteoblasts, bone stromal cells, and activated T cells plays a key role in the process of bone resorption (Xin W, Baudhuin *et al.*, 2013). RANKL binds specifically to the receptor, RANK, is expressed in osteoclast progenitors/ mature osteoclasts. The RANKL-RANK interaction results in the activation of osteoclastogenesis by promoting maturation of osteoclast progenitors into mature osteoclasts. It also inhibits apoptosis of osteoclasts (Gonzalez –Suarez E Dougall *et al.*, 2007; Roodman *et al.*, 2001). RANKL is therefore linked to the resorption of bones. OPG, an anti-inflammatory protein, derived from the osteoblasts and bone stromal cells inhibits osteoclastogenesis. It acts as a soluble decoy recep- tor specific for RANKL (Yasuda *et al.*, 1998). Binding of OPG with RANKL inhibits the RANKL– RANK interaction on the osteoclast cell membranes, thereby inhibiting osteoclastogenesis and subsequent bone loss. Impairment of the fine balance between RANKL and OPG is responsible for the development of osteoporosis either through an increase in RANKL or a decrease in OPG (Fig. 2). Bucay *et al.,* 1998 studied the role of OPG deficiency in OPG-knockout mice generated by the targeted deletion of the *OPG* gene (Bucay *et al.,* 1998). They demonstrated development of an osteoporotic skeletal phenotype, including a high bone-remodeling rate, decreased BMD, and increased incidence of fragility fractures and bone deformities in OPG-knockout mice. These effects stem from the unopposed RANKL activity because of the absence of a decoy receptor. OPG-knockout mice are the first animal model for studying osteoporosis. Therefore, OPG is an important negative regulator of osteoclastogenesis. Another molecule that stimulates osteoclastogenesis is M-CSF. M-CSF increases the number of osteoclast progenitors, and RANKL then binds to its receptor RANK expressed on the surface of osteoclast progenitors (Lacey *et al.,* 1998). Various hormones, growth factors, and cytokines regulate the OPG/ RANK/RANKL axis (Trouvin *et al.,* 2010). Proresorptive cytokines are IL-1, IL-7, IL-17, and tumor necrosis factor-alpha (TNF-α) as they upregulate RANKL, whereas IL-4, IL-13, and interferon-γ are antiresorptive cytokines as they suppress osteoclastogenesis (Trouvin *et al.,* 2010; Theill *et al.,* 2002).

COPD and OPG/RANK/RANKL Axis

Bai *et al.,* studied the level of inflammatory cytokines and OPG/RANK/RANKL protein levels in 80 stable male COPD patients (Bai *et al.,* 2011). They found a significant correlation between radiographic emphysema measured by low-attenuation area (LAA%) and low BMD in COPD patients who are current or former smokers. Compared to COPD patients with normal BMD, patients with low BMD had significantly higher levels of RANKL and a higher RANKL/OPG ratio. The serum levels of IL-6 and TNF-α were also found to be significantly higher in the COPD patients with low BMD, but the level of IL-1β, although higher in the low BMD group than in the normal BMD group, did not reach statistical significance. Cytokines such as IL-6, TNF-α, and IL-1β are secreted by bone stromal cells and monocytes and increase the production of both RANKL and OPG, but their dominant effect is on the RANKL. Eagan *et al.,* also noted significantly lower levels of OPG in

COPD patients compared to the control (Eagan *et al.*, 2010). The characteristics of COPD is the development of systemic inflammation with resulting rise in the serum levels of inflammatory cytokines eg, IL-6, TNF-α, and IL-1β (Marin A,Garcia-Rio *et al.*, 2010; Panda A, Sapey *et al.*, 2009). These cytokines tilt the balance of the OPG/RANK/RANKL axis towards RANKL, which results in the development of osteoporosis in COPD patients. Interestingly, the elevated RANKL can also upregulate the expression of IL-6 and TNF-α, which may augment inflammatory milieu of COPD patients (Theoleyre *et al.*, 2004).

wnt/β-catenin signaling system

Another signaling pathway of importance in osteoporosis is Wnt/ β -catenin signaling system. Wnt/ β -catenin signaling system is one of the main mechanisms controlling osteoblastogenesis (Krishnan *et al.*, 2006). First, Wnt/ β -catenin pathway promotes osteoblastogenesis by stimulating differentiation of pluripotent MSCs toward the osteoblast lineage and decreasing differentiation of MSCs toward adipogenic lineage (Rodda *et al.*, 2006). Second, Wnt signaling promotes osteoblast survival by inhibiting its apoptosis (Zeng X, Almeida *et al.*, 2004). Wnt/ β -catenin signaling system also inhibits the osteoclastogenesis process by stimulating production and secretion of OPG (Duan P, Glass *et al.*, 2016). Therefore, activation of Wnt/ β -catenin signaling pro- motes bone formation, whereas inhibition of Wnt signaling promotes bone resorption and contributes to osteoporosis (Lecarpentier Y, Patel *et al.*, 2002). Kneidinger *et al* analyzed the Wnt/ β -catenin signals in the lung tissues obtained from COPD patients undergoing lung transplantation and reported decreased activity of Wnt/ β -catenin signals in COPD patients. The impaired activity of Wnt/ β-catenin signals may explain the occurrence of both emphysema and osteoporosis (Romme EA, Kneidinger *et al.*, 2013).

p38 MAPK in COPD

COPD is a heterogeneous disorder which includes different clinical and functional phenotypes, sustained by various inflammatory mechanisms (Barnes *et al.*,

2019). Several observations suggest a possible involvement of the mitogen-activated protein kinases (MAPKs) pathway in the COPD-related atrophying process. Within such a complex pathophysiologic context, most subjects with COPD are featured by an inflammatory response largely mediated by neutrophils and macrophages, whereas a minority of patients develop a predominant eosinophilic inflammation (Barnes *et al.,* 2019). With regard to neutrophilic inflammation, key pathogenic roles are played by cigarette smoke, airborne pollutants, oxidative stress, bacteria, and viruses, which activate pro-inflammatory pathways involving pivotal functions exerted by p38 MAPK (Figure 3) (Barnes *et al.,* 2019).

p38 MAPK is activated via a sequential phosphorylation cascade initiated by some upstream MAPK kinase kinases (MAPKKK) such as apoptosis signal-regulating kinase 1 (ASK1) and transforming growth factor-β-activated kinase 1 (TAK1), which phosphorylate MAPK kinases (MAPKK) MKK3 and MKK6 (Chung *et al.,* 2011). The latter in turn catalyze the dual phosphorylation- dependent activation of p38 MAPK, taking place at threonine-180 and tyrosine-182 amino acid residues, respectively (Chung *et al.,* 2011). As a consequence of such a sequential chain of phosphorylations, p38 results to be fully activated, thus becoming able to phosphorylate and activate several substrates. Activation of p38 MAPK signaling module significantly contributes to induction, persistence, and progression of airway inflammation in COPD (Huang *et al.,* 2013). In particular, active p38 phosphorylates histone H3 inside the promoters of genes encoding pro-inflammatory cytokines and chemokines (Figure 4) (Saccani *et al.,* 2002). Through this action p38 facilitates the accessibility of the transcription factor NF-κB (nuclear factor-κB) to its DNA binding sites exposed on phosphorylated and phospho-acetylated promoters (Figure 4), thereby enhancing geneexpression.

In addition to favouring such a transcriptional effect, p38 MAPK also acts at the post- transcriptional level by phosphorylating MAP kinase-activated protein kinase 2 (MAPKAPK2 or MK2). Following p38-dependent activation, MK2 in turn phosphorylates two crucial serine residues (Ser-52 and Ser-178) of tristetraprolin, thus inactivating this regulatory protein which plays a very important anti– inflammatory role via destabilization of multiple mRNAs transcribed from genes coding for several pro-inflammatory mediators (ONeil *et al.*, 2018). Hence, p38 activation results in stabilization of these mRNAs, leading to an increased production of cytokines and chemokines implicated in COPD neutrophilic endotype, including interleukin 1β (IL-1β), interleukin-8 (IL-8) and tumor necrosis factor-α (TNF-α). Therefore, inhibition of p38 MAPK activation potentially represents a suitable anti–inflammatory strategy for COPD treatment (Behrens G, Winzen *et al.*, 2018; Norman *et al.*, 2015).

Role of p38 MAPK activation in COPD pathobiology

In murine models of experimentally induced emphysema, it has been shown that acute and chronic exposure to cigarette smoke up-regulated the activation and expression of p38 MAPK, which stimulated the production of pro-inflammatory cytokines and chemokines, as well as the consequent neutrophilic infiltration of lungs (Marumo *et al.*, 2014). These results are consistent with the findings reported by several human studies, that have documented in COPD patients the presence of high levels of the phosphorylated, active form of p38 MAPK. Indeed, when compared with normal subjects, the expression of phospho-p38α was shown to be significantly increased in macrophages located inside the alveolar spaces of lung surgical specimens removed from COPD patients (Renda *et al.*, 2008). These results werecorroborated by Western blot analysis, showing a marked increase of phospho-p38α expression in cell protein extracts of alveolar macrophage cultures, obtained from COPD patients (Renda *et al.*, 2008). The number of phospho-p38 positive alveolar macrophages resulted to be closely correlated with the impairment of respiratory function, assessed as decreases in both FEV1 (forced expiratory volume in one second) percentage of predicted values and FEV1/FVC (forced vital capacity) ratio (Renda *et al.*, 2008). Moreover, phospho-p38α expression was found to be also enhanced in CD8 + T lymphocytes infiltrating the alveolar walls of COPD patients (Renda *et al.*, 2008) Taken together, these data suggest that activation of p38 MAPK signaling pathway implements an intercellular loop connecting CD8 + T cells and alveolar macrophages, which significantly contributes to the onset and perpetuation of the inflammatory response underlying COPD pathobiology. Indeed, p38 MAPK inhibitors are capable of suppressing the release of pro-inflammatory mediators from alveolar macrophages and other immune/inflammatory cells of patients with COPD (Armstrong *et al.*, 2011). Therefore, MAPK inhibition can potentially attenuate airway chronic inflammation.

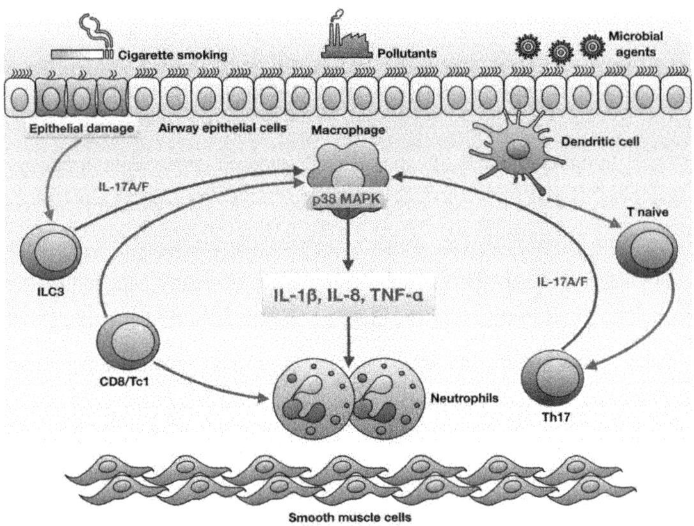

Figure 3. Role of p38 MAPK in COPD pathobiology. Cigarette smoke, airborne pollutants, and microbial agents activate p38 MAPK at the level of alveolar macrophages and other inflammatory cells. As a consequence, p38 signaling pathway induces the release of proinflammatory cytokines and chemokines (IL-1β, IL-8, TNF-α), which together with other mediators (IL-17A and IL-17 F) produced by Th17 and ILC3 cells contribute to recruitment and activation of neutrophils.

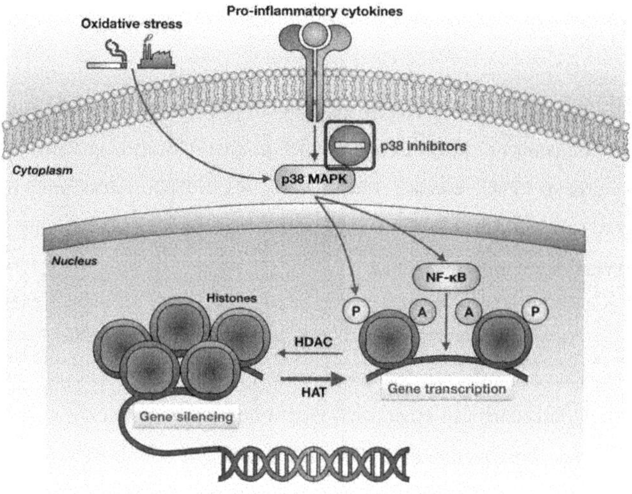

Figure 4. Potential role of p38 MAPK inhibitors in COPD treatment. p38 MAPK inhibitors suppress oxidative stress -induced activation of p38. As a consequence, these drugs inhibit the cellular effects of p38 MAPK, including histone phosphorylation that results in the facilitation of histone acetylation catalyzed by histone acetylases (HAT), which thus overcome the activity of histone deacetylases (HDAC) and promote the access of NFκB to its DNA recognition sites.

In addition to alveolar macrophages and CD8+ T lymphocytes, also small airway epithelial cells from COPD patients express higher levels of phospho-p38 MAPK when compared with nonsmoker controls (Gaffey *et al.*, 2013). It is thus likely that airway epithelial cells contribute to COPD pathogenesis by releasing a wide array of pro-inflammatory mediators as a consequence of the activation of p38 MAPK pathway, induced by various stimuli such as cigarette smoke, airborne pollutants and infectious agents. Consistently with these findings, the expression of phospho-p38

MAPK was reported to be up-regulated in sputum samples of COPD patients (Huang *et al.*, 2013).

Moreover, this increased activation of p38 MAPK remarkably correlated with sputum amounts of neutrophils and IL-8, as well as with lung function impairment, measured as FEV1 decrease (Huang *et al.*, 2013). Such results imply that in COPD p38 MAPK activity is strongly associated with the progression of lung inflammation and respiratory function decline.

Airway inflammation and p38 MAPK activation further intensify during COPD exacerbations. For example, common triggers of COPD exacerbations such as bacterial infections can synergize with pro-inflammatory cytokines like TNF-α, thus enhancing phosphorylation-dependent activation of p38 MAPK (Watanabe *et al.*, 2004). Indeed, when primary cultures of human bronchial epithelial cells were exposed to both TNF-α and non-typeable *Haemophilus influenzae*, phospho-p38 MAPK expression increased, and this amplification of pro-inflammatory signal transduction evoked an up-regulation of IL-8 release from airway epithelial cells (Gallelli *et al.*, 2010). As a consequence, neutrophilic inflammation can worsen because of the powerful chemo attractant action exerted by IL-8 on neutrophils (Chung *et al.*, 2005). Moreover, as a further result of the exposure of bronchial epithelial cells to the synergistic actions of TNF-α and *Haemophilus influenzae*, a p38-MAPK dependent activation of the pro-apoptotic enzyme caspase-3 also occurred (Gallelli *et al.*, 2010). In the same cell cultures, apoptosis was shown to be also elicited via p38-MAPK activa- tion caused by hydrogen peroxide, a common mimicker of the oxidative stress associated with COPD (Pelaia *et al.*, 2004). Therefore, the p38 MAPK signaling pathway is significantly implicated in the induction of airway epithelial damage promoted by several pathogenic factors such as pro-inflammatory cytokines, infectious agents, and oxidative stress. A p38 MAPK-mediate persistent injury of bronchial epithelium thus impairs tissue integrity and favors epithelial permeability to bacteria and viruses, thereby implementing a deleterious self-perpetuating vicious circuit which makes airways more susceptible to the pathogenic actions of various inducers of COPD exacerbations.

Apoptotic mechanisms in the pathogenesis of COPD

Apoptosis

Apoptosis, "normal" or "programmed" cell death, is an evolutionarily conserved, innate process by which cells systematically inactivate, disassemble, and degrade their own structural and functional components. The term "apoptosis" was first introduced by Kerr *et al* in 1972 (Colling RJ Kerr *et al* 1972). It is a key mechanism allowing multicellular animals to tightly regulate cell growth (Baetu and Hiscott 2002). Necrosis, "accidental" cell death, is a pathological process which occurs when cells are exposed to a serious physical or chemical insult. During necrosis loss of membrane integrity leads to the influx of water and extracellular ions. Intracellular organelles, most notably the mitochondria, and the entire cell swell and rupture and the cytoplasmic contents are released into the extracellular fluid. During apoptosis coordinated morphological and biochemical changes occur within the nucleus, cytoplasm, organelles and plasma membrane (Fadok VA, Cohen 1993). Chromatin condenses and aggregates along the nuclear periphery and fragmentation of the nucleus occurs into chromatin containing fragments. Other cytoplasmic organelles remain structurally intact, although pore formation in the mitochondrial membrane is associated with apoptosis. The cell rounds up, dissociates itself from its neighbors and shrinks, throwing out protuberances that separate into membrane-bound "apoptotic bodies", containing cytoplasmic organelles and nuclear material. Within tissues apoptotic bodies are rapidly phagocytosed by neighboring cells (Fadok VA, Cohen 1993).

Table 1.3 Markers upregulating (↑) or downregulating (↓) apoptosis in COPD

	Apoptotic markers	Apoptosis
	bcl-2	↓
	bax	↑
	bad	↑
	Akt	↓
	TNF-α	↑
	Fas–Fas ligand	↑
	p53	↑
	4-Hydroxy-2-nonenal	↑
	sFRP-1	↑

Apoptosis can be triggered through two major pathways, one implicating death receptor ligation and the other the release of cytochrome c from mitochondria (Baetu and Hiscott 2002) (Table 1.3). The death receptor pathway is initiated by the ligation of members of the tumor necrosis factor (TNF) family, such as TNF-α and Fas-ligand, to their respective ligands, TNF receptor 1, and Fas (Baetu and Hiscott 2002). These "death-inducing" receptors recruit the death-inducing signaling complex through interaction with adaptor proteins such as Fas associated death domain protein (FADD). In turn, FADD recruits caspase-8. Caspase-8 activation leads to either direct activation of caspase-3, or to cleaving of Bid, a member of the bcl-2 family, which in turn targets mitochondria for cytochrome c release (Baetu and Hiscott 2002). The mitochondrial pathway can be triggered by both external and internal stimuli. Members of the bcl-2 family of proteins, like bcl-2, bax, and bad, gather at the surface of mitochondria, where they compete to regulate cytochrome c release, which leads to caspase-9 activation. Bcl-2 is an antiapoptotic and bad and bax are proapoptotic members of this family (Baetu and Hiscott 2002). Akt is a serine–threonine kinase that phospholylates and thereby inactivates the proapoptotic proteins bad and caspase 9, and elevates the expression of the antiapoptotic protein bcl-2 (Plataki M, Datta et al 2006). Both pathways converge at the level of caspase-3 activation. Caspases are proteolytic enzymes, the executioners of apoptosis. Caspase activation results in DNA laddering, characteristic of apoptotic cells, and to the cleavage of cytoskeletal proteins. p53 is a critical mediator of two different cellular responses following exposure to DNA damage: growth arrest in the G1 phase of the cell cycle or apoptosis in the case of irreparable damage (Plataki M, Datta,Canman and Kastan 1997). 4-Hydroxy-2-nonenal (4-HNE) is an end-product of lipid peroxidation, which is involved in provoking the toxic effects of oxidative stress to cells, promoting apoptosis (Rabacchi *et al* 2004). The frizzled- related protein sFRP-1 plays a part in the disruption of the normal Wnt signaling status and may also promote the apoptotic process (Plataki M, Jones and Jomary 2002).

Lymphocyte apoptosis in COPD

Studies quantifying the inflammation of the airways in smokers and defining their phenotype found that the predominant inflammatory cell present was the $CD8^+$ T-cell and that their number correlated inversely with the degree of airflow limitation (Saetta *et al* 1993; Jeffery 1998; Hodge, Hodge, Reynolds, *et al* 2003; Hogg *et al* 2004; Chrysofakis *et al* 2004; Tsoumakidou *et al* 2004). These findings suggest an important role for activated T-cells in the pathogenesis of airway abnormalities in COPD. A possible mechanism in order to prevent permanent damage and remodeling in COPD could be removal of excess inflammatory cells, including T-cells, by apoptosis, as has been suggested in other disease models.

Human studies

Hodge, Hodge, Reynolds, *et al* (2003) assessed apoptosis of T lymphocytes isolated from peripheral blood in COPD patients, and found significantly increased apoptosis of stimulated T-cells, CD4, and CD8, compared with controls. There was no significant difference in levels of apoptosis between CD4 and CD8 T-cell subsets in

COPD patients. An upregulation of Fas, TNF-α, TNF receptor 1, and TGF receptor (TGFR) was also observed. Monocyte production of TGF-β and release of active TGF- β in the peripheral blood were increased. There was a decrease in anti-apoptotic bcl2 and IL-7R expression in the peripheral blood T-cells in COPD (Hodge *et al* 2005). The authors concluded that the increased T-cell death may be associated with both an increase in pro-apoptotic and a decrease in anti-apoptotic mediators in the peripheral blood in COPD. The same group investigated apoptosis of lung-derived T-cells (Hodge *et al* 2005). They found an increased percentage and absolute number of apoptotic BAL-derived T-cells in COPD. In addition, there was no significant change in the percentage of T-cells expressing bcl2 or bax, although p53 expression and activated caspases by BAL-derived $CD3^+$ T-cells were significantly increased in COPD (Hodge *et al* 2005).

Pathophysiologic implications

Several observations can be made based on the findings by Hodge, Hodge, Reynolds, *et al* (2003). The increased numbers of T-cells in COPD lungs may result from local proliferation of T-cells in the lung or enhanced trafficking from the bloodstream. This trafficking also occurs from the airways to the bloodstream. Therefore, it is possible that increased apoptosis of T-cells in the peripheral blood in COPD may result either from local apoptotic stimuli in the airways or from apoptotic stimuli in the peripheral blood (Hodge, Hodge, Reynolds, *et al* 2003; Hodge *et al* 2005). Increased numbers of apoptotic T-cells in the lung, if not effectively cleared, may lead to secondary necrosis, which has a pro-inflammatory effect. Furthermore, the increased secretion of TGF-β by monocytes may be attributed to ingestion of increased numbers of apoptotic cells (Fadok *et al* 1998). Increased rates of T-cell apoptosis may lead to a defective immune response to infective organisms, contributing to the high frequency of infections seen in COPD (Hodge *et al* 2005). The decrease in the CD4/CD8 ratio seen in COPD cannot be explained by a preferential increase in the apoptosis of CD4 cells. Recent studies in mice showed that cigarette smoke exposure specifically prevented the expansion and maximal activation of CD4 T-cells and reduced the number of both activated CD4 and CD8 T-cells. Consequently, smoke exposure decreased the activated CD4:CD8 T-cell ratio from 3 to 1.5 (Gary, Robbins *et al* 2004). The mutagenic effect of cigarette smoke on "susceptible" smokers could predispose dendritic cells to production of cytotoxic $CD8^{+}$ cells, which in turn induce epithelial cell death and apoptosis by perforin (Chrysofakis et al 2004; Tzanakis *et al* 2004) (Figure 5).

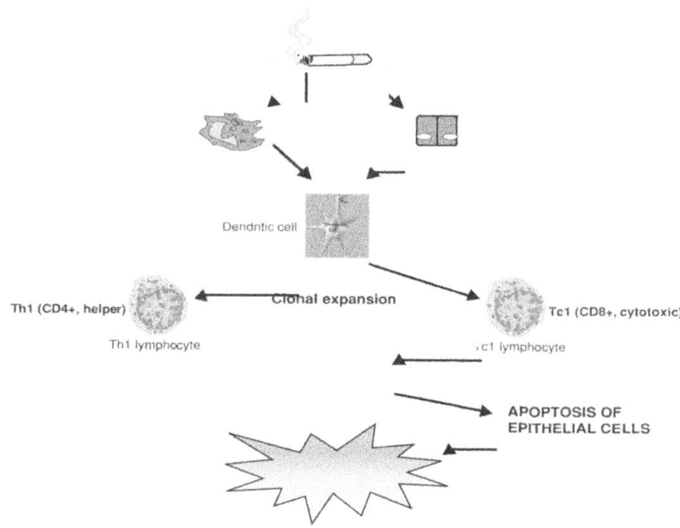

Figure 5 : Oxidative stress of cigarette smoke in "susceptible" smokers activates adaptive immunity, predisposing dendritic cells to clonal expansion of CD4 $^{+}$ and especially of cytotoxic CD8 $^{+}$ cells, inducing epithelial cell death by perforin.

OSTEOCLASTOGENESIS

Osteoclasts are formed by the fusion of mononuclear progenitors of the monocyte macrophage family (Hofbauer LC et al, Teitelbaum 2000) Osteoclasts differentiation is characterized by different features: polynucleation due to cell fusion, formation of ruffled borders for proton enzyme and acid secretion, associated synthesis of vacuolar proton pumps and different enzymes and formation of a sealing zone to prevent enzyme and acid leakage. Tartrate resistant acid phosphatase (TRAP) positive multinucleated cells are formed from mononuclear cells obtained from mouse bone marrow, spleen, thymus, peripheral blood and stromal cells in the presence of 1α,2 dihydroxy vitamin D3 and dexamethasone (Udagawa *et al.,* 1990).

Stromal cells and osteoblasts are essential for osteoclastogenesis as they produce the two essential molecules that are involved in the process of macrophage colony-stimulating factor (M-CSF) and receptor for activation of nuclear factor kappa B ligand (RANKL) (Hofbauer LC et al, Teitelbaum 2000).

RANKL (also known as OPGL and TRANCE) activates mature osteoclasts and regulates osteoclast formation from bone marrow precursors in the presence of M-CSF (Lacey *et al.,* 1998). RANKL is a transmembrane protein found on stromal cells or osteoblasts that binds to either RANK or OPG. It is now known that OPG is a soluble "decoy" receptor that competes with RANK for RANKL (Lacey *et al.,* 1998). The binding of OPG to RANKL inhibits osteoclastogenesis, whereas binding of RANK stimulates it. The balance between OPG and RANKL determines the amount of bone resorbed by controlling the activation of RANK on osteoclasts. Inhibition of RANK by the cell-permeable inhibitory peptide RANK receptor inhibitor (RRI) blocked RANKL-induced osteoclast formation from murine bone marrow macrophages (H. Kim *et al.,* 2009). Multinucleated osteoclasts are highly polarized cells. Different lytic enzymes such as TRAP and pro-Cathepsin K (pro-CATK) are secreted from the highly specialized membrane into the resorption pit (Howship's lacunae). By this process the osteoclast erodes the underlying bone. Degradation products (collagen fragments solubilized phosphate and calcium) are resorbed by the osteoclast, processed and then rereleased to metabolic circulation.

Matrix metalloproteinases (MMPs)

Matrix metalloproteinases (MMPs), a group of calcium-activated zinc ion endopeptidases widely found in a variety of connective tissues, play an essential role in the degradation of the extracellular matrix and basement membrane enzyme. They are differentially expressed during different stages of COPD development (Abd EI – Fatah MF – 2015, Muroski *et al.,* 2008). MMP-9 is produced by osteoclasts and osteoclast precursor cells, the monocytes also. It is essential for recruitment of preosteoclasts into bone and their local migration into the diaphysis (Engsig *et al.*, 2000). Specific expression of MMP-9 in osteoclasts may play an important role in osteoclastic bone resorption, thereby promoting osteoporosis. In contrast, TIMP-1 prevents bone resorption (Hill *et al.,* 1994). The TIMPs are endogenous natural inhibitors of MMPs. The airway MMP-9/TIMP-1 ratio is considered a biomarker of airway tissue destruction and of the dynamic equilibrium of repair (Tanaka *et al.,* 2000).

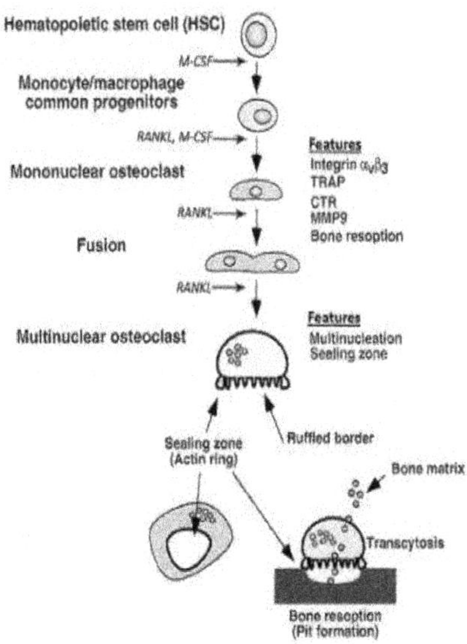

Figure 6. Overview of osteoclastogenesis (Gallo 2008)

TNF-α

TNF-α is a multifaceted cytokine and a well-recognized systemic inflammatory factor related to the occurrence and development of a variety of the systemic complications of COPD, including osteoporosis. TNF-α is also an important regulator of bone metabolism and remodeling. It stimulates osteoclast differentiation in a synergistic manner (McLean *et al.,* 2009). A study by Pinto-Plata showed that levels of the inflammatory markers IL-6 and TNF-α became higher and the levels of markers of injury and repair became lower as the disease progressed (GOLD1 vs. 4) (Pinto *et al.,* 2012). Bon *et al.,* also showed a clear correlation between many serum inflammatory cytokines, including IL-1, IL-6, and TNF-α, and the severity of emphysema as assessed by high-resolution CT (Bon *et al.,* 2009). Levels of IL-1, IL-6, TNF-α, and other cytokines have been shown to stimulate osteoclast differentiation (Mundy *et al.,* 2007). Inflammatory cytokines can also directly act on osteoclasts and their precursor cells, which increases osteoclast activity, causing bone destruction and bone loss (Ragab *et al.,* 2002). In addition, these inflammatory cytokines can interact with the osteoprotegerin (OPG), Members of the receptor activator of NF-kB (RANK) and receptor activator of NF-kB ligand (RANKL) and osteoprotegerin (OPG) system are critical in bone homeostasis through regulation of osteoclasts (Lehouck *et al.,* 2011; Calikoglu M , Kwan *et al.,* 2004). OPG is an endogenous receptor antagonist of RANKL. It blocks the binding of RANKL to RANK, so inhibiting osteoclast development and bone resorption. RANKL and OPG are the promoting and inhibitory factors of osteoclast differentiation, respectively. They maintain a certain ratio within the body. Imbalances in this ratio can disrupt bone metabolism, leading to reduced bone mass/osteoporosis among other bone diseases (McLean *et al.,* 2009; Calikoglu M ,Kwan *et al.,* 2004; Simonet *et al.,* 1997).

In COPD patients with osteoporosis, the blood level of soluble RANKL and the ratio of RANKL/OPG were increased and associated inversely with bone mineral density (BMD), suggesting that the disturbance of the RANKL/RANK pathway, probably by interaction with systemic inflammation, is involved in bone loss in

COPD. Membrane-bound RANKL (mRANKL) was expressed by a variety of immune cells, including T lymphocytes and neutrophils. In chronic inflammation, expression of mRANKL by neutrophils was upregulated, and RANKL-expressing neutrophils can induce osteoclastogenesis by direct cell contact with osteoclasts (Bai *et al.*, 2011; Chakravarti *et al.*, 2009). Given that neutrophils are the predominant effector cells in airway inflammation and lung destruction, and that there is evidence of systemic activation of neutrophils in COPD (Hoenderdos *et al.*, 2013).

RANKL/RANK signaling

The binding of RANKL to the extracellular RANK domain leads to RANK oligomerization and initiation of a series of signaling pathways essential for the differentiation and activation of osteoclasts. The initial step in RANK signaling is formation of a complex with the TNF receptor-associated factor (TRAF) adaptor proteins through the cytoplasmic domain of RANK. Among the six members of the TRAF family, only TRAF6 appears to be critical to osteoclast differentiation and activation (Armstrong *et al.*, 2002; H. H. Kim *et al.*, 1999). RANKL stimulation results in rapid activation of NF-κB signaling, as well as the mitogen-activated protein kinases (MAPK) cascades such as extracellular-signal regulated kinase (ERK), Jun-N terminal kinase (JNK), and p38 stress kinase pathway. Similar to TRAF6, NF-κB is critical for osteoclastogenesis (Iotsova *et al.*,1997). The classic NF-κB signaling pathway involves activation of the IκB kinase (IKK) complex that phosphorylates the IκBs and targets them to ubiquitin dependent degradation (Ghosh and Karin 2002). Events leading to NF-κB activation via TRAF6 include the serine/threonine kinase TAK1 (TGFβ activated kinase 1), TAK1 binding protein 2 (TAB2), phosphorylation of the NF-κB inducing kinase (NIK) and IκB kinases (IKKs) (Theoleyre *et al.*, 2004). p38 is another MAPK involved in mediating key signals induced by RANKL (Li *et al.*, 2002; Matsumoto *et al.*, 2000). The stimulation of p38 results in the downstream activation of the transcription factor MITF (Mansky *et al.*, 2002), which is critical for multinuclear osteoclast formation and osteoclast specific gene expression.

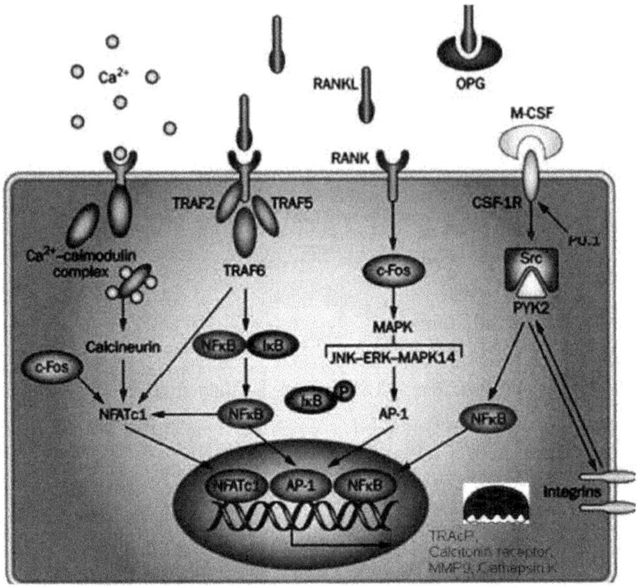

Figure 7 : RANK-dependent intracellular signaling pathways in osteoclast (Edwards and Mundy 2011).

Diagnosis

COPD is heterogeneous, no single diagnostic test can confirm the occurrence of the disease, usually it is diagnosed using spirometry which measures the amount of air that a lung can accommodate and how fast, air is blown out of the lung, additional tests are done to discard the possibility of asthma or heart failure, this include other lung functioning tests such as Methacholine challenge test, a chest X- ray or CT scan and Arterial blood gas analysis which measure the efficiency of the lungs to engage oxygen into the blood and remove carbon dioxide from the blood. Airflow obstruction can be explained as a decreased FEV1/FVC ratio (where FEV1 is forced expired volume in 1 second and FVC is forced vital capacity), i.e., FEV1/FVC is less than 0.7.

Assessment and classification of COPD

The classification is based on the measure of severity of the airflow obstruction interpreted from the guidelines of Global Strategy for the Diagnosis, Management and Prevention of COPD (GOLD).

Table 1.4. Classification of COPD

STAGES	FEV1 %	Post-bronchodilator FEV1/FVC
Mild	≥80%*	<0.7
Moderate	50-79%	<0.7
Severe	30-49%	<0.7
Very severe	<30% or <50% and respiratory failure**	<0.7

*Diagnosis for COPD is done only in case of difficulty in respiration is observed, e.g. cough or troubled breathing. ** If the arterial partial pressure of oxygen is <8.0 kPa (60mm Hg) along with or without arterial partial pressure of carbon dioxide at >6.7 kPa (50mm Hg) while breathing air at sea level.

COPD comorbidities

COPD comorbidities is a rather broad heterogeneous term, including diseases that independently coexist with COPD with no other causation, diseases that share common risk factors and pathogenetic pathways with COPD, diseases that are complicated by the interaction with the lung, and systemic manifestations of COPD, and vice versa. Most commonly COPD is associated with lung cancer and other cancers, asthma, obstructive sleep apnea syndrome, hypertension, cardiovascular disease, diabetes, metabolic syndrome, dysfunctional skeletal myopathies, osteoporosis, and mental disorders. Divo et al in a recent report concluded that lung, pancreatic, esophageal, and breast cancers (the last only for female patients), pulmonary fibrosis, atrial fibrillation/flutter, congestive heart failure, coronary artery disease, gastric/duodenal ulcers, liver cirrhosis, diabetes with neuropathy, and anxiety are the most significant and frequent comorbidities (Divo *et al.*, 2012).

Respiratory comorbidities

Asthma

Both asthma and COPD are major chronic obstructive airway diseases that involve underlying airway inflammation. COPD is characterized by airflow limitation that is not fully reversible, is usually progressive, and is associated with an abnormal inflammatory response of the lungs to noxious particles or gases. Individuals with asthma who are exposed to noxious agents (particularly cigarette smoking) may develop fixed airflow limitation and a mixture of "asthma-like" inflammation and "COPD-like" inflammation. Thus, even though asthma can usually be distinguished from COPD, in some individuals who develop chronic respiratory symptoms and fixed airflow limitation, it may be difficult to differentiate the two diseases. Coexistence of asthma and COPD in elderly patients is often diagnosed (Soriano *et al.*, 2005). In some studies, the overlap diagnosis of asthma and COPD exceeds half of the patients examined (Fu *et al.*, 2014; Marsh *et al.*, 2008). The overlap is identified by finding increased variability of airflow in patients with incompletely reversible airway obstruction (Gibson *et al.*, 2009). The presence of COPD-asthma overlap syndrome is associated with impaired quality of life and more frequent and severe exacerbations compared with COPD only patients (Hardin *et al.*, 2011) .

Lung cancer

COPD patients run an increased risk of developing lung cancer. It is also a factor that contributes to poorer outcomes in lung cancer patients (Global Initiative for Asthma, ACOS, 2014; Kiri *et al.*, 2010). The prevalence of COPD among patients with lung cancer varies from 40% to 70% (Tammemagi *et al.*, 2003; Hashimoto N,

Loganathan *et al.*, 2006). Several reports confirmed that lung cancer occurs in COPD patients late in the natural course of the disease. The prevalence of moderate-to-very severe disease (GOLD stages II–IV) among lung cancer patients reaches 50%, in contrast with only 8% of smokers without lung cancer (Global Initiative for Asthma, ACOS, 2014). The annual incidence of lung cancer is four times higher in COPD patients when compared with the general population (Young *et al.*, 2009).20,24 Three-year survival in patients with COPD and lung cancer has been found to be around 15%, compared with 26% for lung cancer patients without COPD (Global Initiative for Asthma, ACOS ,2014).

Hypertension

Hypertension is very common in COPD patients, but is not associated with increased mortality (Divo *et al.*, 2012). Hypertension is related to the increased systemic inflammation observed in COPD and is correlated with higher Medical Research Council dyspnea scores, reduced capacity for physical activity and airflow obstruction (Schonhofer *et al.*, 1998; Miller *et al.*,2013).

Coronary heart disease

COPD and coronary heart disease share a common major risk factor, which is smoking. The coexistence has been reported to be as high as 30% or even higher in COPD patients. In some studies of the medical records of COPD patients, undiagnosed cases of coronary heart disease reach 70% (Sin *et al.*, 2008). Both diseases are characterized by chronic sustained inflammation and coagulopathy. The key mediator of this sustained inflammation in COPD is probably elevated C-reactive protein levels, which not only maintain bronchial constriction but also increase the risk for coronary disease (Young *et al.*, 2009; Brekke *et al.*, 2008).

Metabolic comorbidities

Diabetes and metabolic syndrome

Diabetes has been reported in several studies to be a frequent COPD comorbidity, with a prevalence as high as 18.7% among COPD patients (Crisafulli *et al.,* 2015). The prevalence of metabolic syndrome is reported to be up to 22.5% in COPD patients. COPD patients have a relatively increased risk of developing diabetes, but also diabetes often presents before diagnosis of COPD, and diabetic patients have an increased risk of developing COPD (Rogliani P, Cazzola *et al.,* 2014; Mannino *et al.,* 2008; Song *et al.,* 2010). This side-by-side development of both diseases is a result of common risk factors, like smoking, and also the synergic effect of systemic inflammation mediated by common cytokines (Tkacova *et al.,* 2010). Diabetes worsens the outcomes of COPD by affecting a number of parameters: shortening time to first hospitalization and increasing hospitalization time and risk of death during exacerbations, increasing Medical Research Council dyspnea scores, and reducing six-minute walking distance. 30 Diabetes worsens 5-year mortality in COPD patients (Fabbri *et al.,* 2008).

COPD and osteoporosis

M-CSF is responsible for both the proliferation and differentiation of osteoclast progenitors (D M Biskobing *et al.,* 1995). RANKL / ODF/ TRANCE / OPGL is a ~35 kDa, membrane-bound signal transducer of the TNF super family responsible for the formation, differentiation and maintenance of osteoclasts (Lacey *et al.,* 1998). Stromal cells and osteoblasts produce two key molecules namely macrophage colony-stimulating factor (M-CSF) and receptor for activation of nuclear factor kappa B ligand (RANKL) that drives osteoclastogenesis (Hofbauer LC, Teitelbaum 2000)

Multiple studies declare that the monocytes and macrophages that express the surface marker CD14 can be differentiated into bone-resorbing osteoclasts (Massey and Flanagan 1999; Takeshita *et al.,* 2000). A separate study by Battaglino *et al.,*

(2002) provide evidence that shows monocyte-macrophage cell lines form osteoclast-like cells that are capable of bone resorption *in vitro* and also report that c-myc is a downstream target of RANKL and its expression is required for RANKL-induced osteoclastogenesis. A study in which MMP level is measured in 70 clinically stable COPD patients and reported that the circulating levels of MMP-9 in patients with COPD is increased compared with the healthy controls (Hill *et al.,* 1994).

Peripheral monocytes from patients with COPD who lose weight had an increased ability to produce TNF-α (de Godoy *et al.,* 1996). Aldonyte *et al.,* (2003) found that LPS stimulated secretion of pro- inflammatory molecules from circulating monocytes differ between healthy and COPD patients. CC-16, an anti-inflammatory protein which plays a protective role against the oxidative stress found low in serum and broncho alveolar lavage (BAL) fluid in chronic lung disorders caused by tobacco smoke and COPD patients respectively. (Broeckaert *et al.,* 2000).

Meta-analysis by Gan (2004) revealed that inflammatory markers like C-reactive protein (CRP), fibrinogen, leucocytes, TNF-α are raised in COPD patients. Levels of protein carbonylation and nitration, lipid peroxidation, and protein oxidation are elevated in blood of COPD patients due to the oxidative stress caused by the cigarette smoke which is known to induce modification to proteins, lipids, and DNA. (Couillard and Prefaut 2005).

An increase in parathyroid hormone (PTH) with low vitamin D levels results in the mobilization of calcium from the bone compartment through bone resorption characterized by the increased osteoclastogenesis (Baldock *et al.,* 2006). Later it was reported that vitamin D deficiency may be responsible for the hyperparathyroidism in COPD patients. PTH was identified to upregulate the IL-18 cytokine which involves in the pro-bone resorptive signaling (Raggatt *et al.,* 2008). Leukocyte-derived IL-1α and TNF-α stimulate bone resorption and IL-6 stimulates the formation of osteoclasts (Ionescu and Schoon 2003).

Barnes (2008) reported that COPD inflammation became resistance to the anti-inflammatory effects of the corticosteroids, even at high doses, as the inflammation progress. This is due to the increased acetylation of the glucocorticoid receptors as the deacetylation of these receptors is blocked due to the reduction in histone deacetylase 2 (HDAC2) levels as a result of oxidative and nitrative stress, thereby preventing it from inhibiting NF-κB-driven inflammation.

Serum levels of 1-CTP, a marker for bone resorption shows a positive correlation to TNF-α receptor II and negatively correlated with the recent weight change in patients with advanced COPD (Førli *et al.,* 2008). MMPs are produced by osteoclasts and osteoclast progenitors, as well as by monocytes/ macrophages. MMPs stimulate osteoclastic bone resorption and promote osteoporosis. In contrast, Tissue inhibitor of metalloproteinases (TIMPs) prevent bone loss (Bolton *et al.,* 2009).

Pro-resorptive cytokines are IL-1, IL-7, IL-17, and tumor necrosis factor-alpha (TNF-α) as they upregulate RANKL, whereas IL-4, IL-13, and interferon-γ are anti-resorptive cytokines as they suppress osteoclastogenesis (Theill *et al.,* 2002; Trouvin and Goeb 2010).

Testosterone (normally increase the BMD), was found low in COPD patients which may indicate the risk for osteoporosis in COPD patients, and low oestrogen concentration are associated with osteoporosis, this support the fact that hypogonadism is a risk factor for osteoporosis (Lehouck *et al.,* 2011).

Lehouck (2011) analysed and reported that the risk factors for COPD such as age, smoking, vitamin D deficiency, low BMD, weight loss, systemic inflammation coincide with that of Osteoporosis.

Cytokines such as IL-6, TNF-α, and IL-1β are secreted by bone stromal cells and monocytes and increase the production of both RANKL and OPG, but their dominant effect is on the RANKL (Bai *et al.,* 2011). MMP-9 and MMP-12 levels are increased and Clara cell protein (CC-16) is reduced in the COPD patients. Previous tuberculosis, asthma (childhood), alpha1- antitrypsin deficiency due to genetic cause and respiratory infections are proved to be a risk factor for COPD . In addition, mice with a loss of MMP-12 were resistant to smoke-induced emphysema, and did not demonstrate any increase in lung inflammation and in the destruction of alveolar walls after smoke exposure (Hautamaki *et al.,* 2004). The mechanism for the abnormal development of the structural changes in the lung extracellular matrix implicates members of serine- and cysteine-protease families and matrix metalloproteases (Carrell *et al.,* 2002; Buhling *et al.,* 2004; Imai *et al.,* 2001). Their dysregulated activity likely causes the pathological disruption of pulmonary collagen and elastin leading to emphysema (Sharafkhaneh *et al.,* 2008). Genetically modified mouse models overexpressing these proteases spontaneously developed emphysema (DArmiento *et al.,* 1992; Churg *et al.,* 2005). Transgenic mice expressing human MMP-1 developed alterations in the lung architecture, as well as emphysematous changes due to the digestion of type III collagen (Shiomi *et al.,* 2003).

Abu-Bakr *et al.,* (2014) observed that PTH was significantly increased, corrected calcium was significantly decreased, and alkaline phosphatase was non-significantly increased in COPD patients and found a negative association of PTH with BMD.

Levels of TNF-α, its receptor, IL-1β, IL-6, Il-8, IL-8, and acute phase reactants are increased in the serum of COPD. Low testosterone levels are associated with osteoporosis and vitamin D concentration in plasma is positively correlated with the BMD (Cielen *et al.,* 2014).

Cathepsin K

SaneShige S 2002, Tezuka *et al.,* (1994) first suggested that cathepsin K may play an important role in osteoclastic bone resorption. Later, it is proved true, as cathepsin K antisense oligodeoxynucleotide inhibit the osteoclastic bone resorption *in vitro* (Inui *et al.,* 1997) and cathepsin K knockout mice exhibit a phenotype of osteopetrosis (Gowen *et al.,* 1999; Saftig *et al.,* 2002). Induced overexpression of the inflammatory cytokine IL-13 in murine lungs stimulated the expression of MMPs and cathepsins, which resulted in emphysematous changes in the lung (Zheng *et al.*, 2000).

NFATc1

NFATc was found to be induced and activated by RANKL during osteoclastogenesis in a TRAF6, c-fos and calcineurin dependent manner. Surprisingly over-expression of NFATc isoforms, NFATc 1 or 2 promoted the differentiation of osteoclast precursor cells into multinucleated osteoclast-like cells even in the absence of RANKL (Ikeda et al 2004). The essential role of NFATc1 in osteoclastogenesis was revealed by the observations that NFATc1 deficient embryonic stem cells cannot differentiate into osteoclasts.

TRAF6

TRAF6 binds to a unique motif located within the membrane proximal region of RANK (Darnay *et al.*, 1999). Among all the TRAF knockout studies, only TRAF6-deficient mice displayed bone abnormalities in that they developed osteopetrosis due to a defect in osteoclastogenesis (Naito *et al.*, 1999, 2002)

AP-1

AP-1 is a dimeric transcription factor composed of members of the Jun proteins (c-Jun, JunB, JunD); the Fos proteins (c-fos, Fra-1, Fra-2, FosB); and ATF proteins. The most common form of AP-1 is composed of c-Jun and c-fos. The lack of c-fos results in pleiotropic defects, including osteopetrosis due to the absence of osteoclasts (Grigoriadis *et al.*, 1994; Johnson *et al.*, 1992). c-fos as well as c-Jun proteins gradually accumulate upon RANKL signalling (Ito *et al.*, 2005). Fra1 together with a dimerization partner different from Jun proteins can rescue osteoclast differentiation in c-Fos-deficient precursors (Bakiri *et al.*, 2007).

SCOPE OF THE STUDY

Chronic obstructive pulmonary disease (COPD) is a preventable yet incurable major public health concern across the world and in the recent decade there has been increased prevalence and mortality among the COPD subjects. By 2012, COPD has been reported to rank as the third leading cause of death by killing more than 3 million people worldwide. This disease progressively decreases breathing capacity and thereby damages the ability to perform daily activities and leads to premature mortality.

India has been known to be adversely affected by COPD and crude estimation suggests that there could be around 30 million COPD subjects in India and this could contribute to the higher percentage of COPD mortality worldwide. This mammoth number of affected subjects has the capability to undermine the state economies and health systems.

Osteoporosis has been determined to be a prinicipal and the most common co-morbid disease of COPD patients. Several risk factors like vitamind deficiency, systemic inflammation and the use of corticosteroids trigger the development of COPD mediated osteoporosis. Both of these diseases impair daily activities of COPD patients and decrease the quality of life. Several studies have implicated the relationship between the prevalence of osteoporosis in COPD subjects yet molecular link and the relationship with the severity of COPD and osteoporosis are obscure.

Understanding the significance of osteoporosis development in COPD and unraveling their molecular mechanisms remains essential. Hence, this study investigates the potential involvement of MAPK and NF-κB pathways in the development of osteoclasts from mild to severe COPD condition

HYPOTHESIS

In this study, it was hypothesized that the preferential secondary osteoporosis development from COPD may be due to the imbalance in various signaling cascades that includes the increased production of monocytes, higher osteoclastogenic factors, altered MAPK signaling and deficit in apoptosis of osteoclasts.

Using peripheral blood mononuclear cells (PBMCs) isolated from blood of COPD and healthy subjects, the present study demonstrated that the osteoclast development and osteoporosis increases with the severity of the disease.

OBJECTIVE

To characterize the molecular mechanisms and key cellular mediators involved in COPD – induced osteoclast activation and bone resorption.

MATERIALS & METHODS

EXPERIMENTAL DESIGN

Whole Blood samples collected from healthy subjects and subjects suffering from Chronic Obstructive Pulmonary Diseases (COPD) were grouped as follows:

Group 1: Healthy Control (n=10).

Group 2: Mild COPD (n=8)

Group 3: Moderate COPD (n=9)

Group 4: Severe COPD (n=13)

Group 5: Very severe COPD (n=11)

Study subjects

Study subjects were recruited from in/out-patients of ESI Hospital, Chennai, India. Ethical approval was obtained from the same institute. Written informed consent was obtained from the study subjects before collecting samples.

Chronic obstructive pulmonary disease (COPD) subjects were selected based on previous history of the disease. Demographic and anthropometric details like age, height, weight, duration of COPD, and medical history of the study objectives were obtained from their medical records of the study subjects. In this study, 41 chronic obstructive pulmonary disease (COPD) subjects with varying severity and 10 normal healthy subjects were recruited. Subjects who had ailments that are not influencing bone metabolism were included in the study. Patients with conditions that influence bone turnover or had taken oral bisphosphonates / TZDs or subjects who were on calcium/estrogen treatment, and subjects with complications like cancer, cirrhosis, osteoporosis etc. were excluded from the study.

Reagents

Recombinant human M-CSF and RANKL, fetal bovine serum (FBS) were purchased from Sigma-Aldrich (St. Louis MO USA). Alpha minimum essential medium (α -MEM), antibiotic-antimycotic solution (100X) were obtained from Invitrogen (Carlsbad, CA). Leucocyte specific tartrate-resistant acid phosphatase (TRAP) kit, L-glutamine and dexamethasone were obtained from Sigma-Aldrich (Germany). Primary antibodies namely Fra1, NFATc1, c-fos, TRAF6, and secondary anti-mouse for NFATc1 and Fra1 whereas secondary anti-rabbit for c-fos and TRAF6 were purchased from Santacruz Biotech Inc. iScript™. Reagent kits for MAPK proteins (ERK, p^{38}, JNK pJNK, B-activing and Aaoptotic proteins (Bcl-2, Bcl-xl, Bax, Caspase-3 and Caspase-9) were also purchased from Santacruz Biotech Inc. iScript^{TM}. cDNA Synthesis Kit from Bio-rad (USA) for cDNA synthesis. Cathepsin k and calcitonin receptor primer from Eurofins genomics (India). RIPA buffer from Thermo scientific (USA) for protein isolation. Pierce BCA Protein Assay Kit, Thermo Scientific (USA) for protein estimation. Cell culture pre-treated 24 well and 96 well were purchased from SPL Life Sciences (Korea) and Nest Biotech (China). Arsenazo III kit for calcium estimation and C-Reactive protein kit (Turbidimetry) for the CRP estimation and hormone kits (PTH, Estrodiol, Testosterone, Vit-D) were also purchased.

Blood and Serum biochemistry

10 ml of peripheral whole blood were drawn from the study participants. 3 ml whole blood was used to carry out biochemical assays. Serum levels of testosterone/17-β estradiol, Parathyroid hormone (PTH), vitamin D were determined using ADVIA Centaur CP Immunoassay System (Siemens Healthcare GmbH) by Chemiluminescence Immuno assay method and Calcium (Arsenazo III method is used using Spectrophotometry at 650 nm,) C- Reactive Protein (measured by Turbidimetry method using Spectrophotometry at 540 nm using BS-400 Chemistry Analyzer (Mindray, China). BMI is calculated using the subjects' height, weight and age.

Measurement of pro-inflammatory cytokines by ELISA

ELISA kits (R&D Systems, Inc) were used to analyze the levels of IL-1β, IL-6, and TNF-α in the osteoclast culture medium in all the four groups and pro-inflammatory cytokines determined based on the manufacturer's directions.

Isolation of mononuclear cells from whole blood

Whole blood samples were diluted in 1:1 with phosphate buffered saline (PBS, without Ca2+ and Mg2+). Diluted blood was layered on top of ficoll in 2:1 ratio and centrifuged at 1800 rpm, for 30 min at room temperature. The cell layer on top of the Ficoll-Paque was collected, resuspended in phosphate buffered saline and centrifuged at 1500 rpm for 10 min for three times to get purified cells (Susa *et al.*, 2004). Subsequently, cells were counted in a hemocytometer and used immediately for surface marker analysis.

Monocytes separation from PBMC by adherence method

Isolated PBMC are cultured in the DMEM medium with 5% FBS for 3 to 4 hrs., allowing the monocytes to adhere to the well surfaces. The lymphocytes are non-adherent cells which can be removed by washing, leaving the monocytes adhered to the surfaces. Then the wells containing adherent cells (monocytes) are cultured with fresh DMEM medium with 5% FBS for 24hrs.

Generation and differentiation of human primary osteoclasts

Whole population of mononuclear cells were cultured in 24 well plate (1×10^6 cells per plate) in 1ml α- minimal essential medium (MEM)) containing pen-strep and 10% FBS and allowed to adhere overnight. After overnight, the medium was semi depleted and replaced with fresh osteoclastogenic differentiation medium containing 25ng/ml MCSF, 40 ng/ml RANKL and 1 μM dexamethasone and 2mM L-glutamine. The cells were re-fed every three days by semi-depletion. On 14th day they were stained for Tartrate Resistant Acid Phosphatase (TRAP), activity using Napthol AS-

BI phosphate and Fast Garnet in the presence of sodium tartrate, as instructed by the manufacturer. The number of TRAP positive, multinucleated (3 or more nuclei) cells were counted in triplicate manner (Henriksen *et al.*, 2012).

Tartrate-resistant acid phosphatase (TRAP) staining

Cells were washed with PBS and fixed with 37% formaldehyde for 30 sec. After washing with PBS, cells were incubated with 0.1% Triton X-100 for 10 min. Cells were washed and then incubated for 60 min at 37°C in dark room with the mixture of solutions containing Fast Garnet GBC, sodium nitrite, Napthol AS-BI phosphoric acid, acetate, and Tartrate of the Leukocyte Acid Phosphatase Assay kit following the manufacturer's instructions. Counter staining was done for 2 min with hamatoxylin solution. Cells were then washed with water gently and TRAP-positive multinucleated cells containing three or more nuclei were considered as osteoclasts.

Measurement of Pro-inflamattory cytokines

ELISA kits (RND systems, Inc.) were used to analyse the levels of Pro inflamattory cytokines (IL-1β, IL-6 and TN-α) (Fig.5.3) in the osteoclast culture medium for all the five groups were determined as per the instructions of the manufacturer.

RNA extraction and reverse transcription – Polymerase chain reaction (RT-PCR) Isolation of RNA from osteoclast cells

After 14 days of culture, the cells were washed with PBS and 1ml trizol reagent was added to the cells at room temperature for 10 min. Then, chloroform was added and centrifuged at 10,000 rpm for 10 min. The aqueous phase formed was removed and the RNA was precipitated by adding isopropanol. This mixture was centrifuged at 12,000 rpm for 30 min. Pellet was collected, stored at – 80°C. The quantity and the integrity of the isolated RNA was assessed by optical density measurements, obtaining the ratio of absorbance values at 260nm and 280nm using a Bio-photometer (Eppendorf, Germany).

cDNA synthesis:

Total RNA (1μg) was reverse-transcribed into cDNA by using iScript™ cDNA Synthesis Kit (Bio-rad) following exactly manufactures guidelines.

Table 4.1. cDNA reaction mix

Components	Volume (μl)
5x iScript select reaction mix	4
Oligo(dT) 20 primer or random primer	2
RNA sample (1 μg of total RNA)	Variable
iScript reverse transcriptase	1
Nuclease-free water	Variable
Total	20

Incubate the reaction mix at following PCR condition:

5 minutes at 25°C

30 minutes at 42°C

5 minutes at 85°C

Hold at 4°C.

Then, the cDNA was stored at -80°C.

Polymerase chain reaction

Table 4.2. PCR reaction mix

Components	Volume (μl)
PCR master mix	8
Forward primer	1
Reverse primer	1
cDNA template	2
Sterile milli Q water	8
Total	20

Table 4.3. Primer details

Target gene	Primer sequences	Product Size (bp)
cathepsin K	F 5'-CCGCAGTAATGACACCCTTT-3' R 5'-AAGGCATTGGTCATGTAGCC-3'	258
β-actin	F 5' TCACCCACACTGTGCCCATCTACGA3' R 5'CAGCGGAACCGCTCATTGCCAATGG3'	285

PCR amplifications were performed as follows: 30 cycles for cathepsin K (94°C for 1 minute, 60°C for 1 minute, and 72°C for 1 minute) and 30 cycles for β-actin (94°C for 35 s, 64°C for 45 s, and 72°C for 1 minute). RT-PCR of β-actin was used as an endogenous control. PCR products were visualized on 1.8% agarose gels stained with ethidium bromide and analyzed by densitometry (da Gloria Carvalho *et al.*, 2010). Data are presented as the relative expression of cathepsin K to the β-actin corresponding to individual sample and analyzed with image lab software (Bio Rad, USA) (Fig.5.5).

Western blot analysis

Isolation of proteins from osteoclasts:

Osteoclasts derived from PBMCs after 14 days of incubation with RANKL and M-CSF medium were discarded gently and rinsed with PBS and suspended with RIPA buffer containing protease inhibitors (0.155M Tris-HCl, pH 7.2, 0.155mM ammonium chloride, 0.1M KCl, 0.1% NP-40, 0.1mM EDTA). Incubation was done on a rotating shaker for 10 min at 4°C. Cells were centrifuged for 10min at 12,000 rpm and incubated in ice for 30 min at -20°C and the supernatants were collected and stored at -80°C until required.

Determination of protein concentration:

The protein concentration was determined (Eppendorf, Germany) using the BCA protein assay Kit (Thermo Scientific). The working reagent was prepared by mixing 50 parts of reagent A (Bicinchoninic acid, Sodium carbonate, Sodium tartrate and Sodium bicarbonate) and 1 part of reagent B (Copper sulphate pentahydrate) according to protocol. 1000 µl of BCA reagent was added to 5 µl of sample in the micro centrifuge tube and incubated for one hour at 37°C. The tube was then cooled to room temperature and the absorbance was measured at 562nm (Eppendorf, Germany).

SDS-polyacrylamide gel electrophoresis (SDS-PAGE)

Proteins were separated on discontinuous polyacrylamide gel electrophoresis. The upper stacking gel (5%) was composed of 0.5 M Tris-HCl (pH 6.8), 10 % SDS, 10% APS, 29:1 acrylamide-bisacrylamide. The lower resolving gel (10%) was composed of 1.5M Tris-HCl (pH 8.8), 10% SDS, 10% APS, 29:1 acrylamide-bisacrylamide. Proteins were resuspended in SDS sample buffer (0.125 M Tris-HCl, pH 6.8; 20% glycerol; 10% SDS; 0.2M DTT; 0.02% Bromophenol blue; prepared as 2X stock), mixed thoroughly and incubated for 5 min. at 90°C. Protein samples were loaded and allowed to run along the running buffer (25 mM Tris, 192 mM glycine, 0.1% SDS, 20% methanol) at 80V until the samples entered the resolving gel and then it was set at 100 V (Hames 1998) .

Immunoblotting

Proteins separated via SDS-PAGE were transferred onto a PVDF membrane (Santacruiz) using wet blot in the transfer buffer (25 mM Tris, 192 mM glycine, 20% methanol) (Ni *et al.*, 2016) for 45 minutes at 100v. The membranes were blocked in the TBS (50 mM Tris- HCl, pH 7.4; 150 mM NaCl) containing 5% dry milk at room temperature for 120 minutes. The membranes were then incubated with appropriate antibodies (c-Fos 1:1000, NFATc1 1:1000) at room temperature for overnight in TBS containing 3% BSA. Similarly MAPK – pathway proteins, ERK, PERK, p^{38}, pp^{38}, JNK, PJNK and apoptotic proteins – Pro (Bax, Caspase – 3 and Caspase – 9) anti (Bcl-2 and Bcl-xl) were also incubated with appropriate primary and secondary antibodies at room temperature for ovr night in TBS containing 3% BSA.

Following antibody incubation, the membranes were washed 3 times (each 5 min) using TBS and TBST (TBS containing 0.1% tween-20). After washing it was incubated with secondary conjugated anti- rabbit (c-Fos, TRAF6) and anti-mouse (NFATc1, Fra1) at a ratio of 1:5000 for 60 min at room temperature.

The membrane were washed with TBS and TBST for 3 times (each 5 min). The visualization of immunoreactivity was achieved using ECL plus detection kit. Solution A and B (ECL) were mixed into 1:1 ratio (each 250 μl) and incubate for 2-3 min at room temperature. The excess detection reagent was drained from the membrane. The signals were visualized by enhanced chemiluminescence (Pierce, Rockford, IL). The protein concentrations were normalized to β- actin levels.

RESULTS

5.1 Blood and Serum biochemistry

The baseline clinical and biochemical characteristics of the study groups are shown in table 5.1.

Table 5.1. Baseline characteristics of the study subjects.

Variables	Control	Mild COPD	Moderate COPD	Severe COPD	Very severe COPD
No of subjects (Female/ Male)	10 (6/4)	8(4/4)	9(5/4)	13(8/5)	11(6/5)
Age (years)	46.24±6.3	48.73±5.2	47.9±4.9	52.48±3.8 c**	51.75±5.6 d*
Vitamin D (ng/ml)	54.5±10	32.78±5.1 a***	19.08±4.4 b***	7.35±1.8 c***	3.5±2.3 d***
PTH (pg/ml)	67.06±2.6	70.2 ± 3.2 a*	67.7 ± 2.6	71.6 ± 3.4 c**	78.3 ± 5.9 d***
BMI kg/cm2	25.5±2.6	24.6±3.1	24.3±2.5	21.63±2.1 c***	20.1±2.4 d***
Testosterone (ng/ml)	5.35 ± 2.81	3.4±1.09	2.4±1.7	2.36±1.6	2.35±0.96 d*
Estradiol (pg/L)	22.75 ± 1.38	19.37±0.98 a**	18.61±1.92 b**	17.61±1. 83 c***	15.20±1.2 d***
Calcium (mg/dL)	8.32±0.09	7.21±0.65 a***	7.64±0.97 b***	8.25±0.64 c***	10.25±0.8 d***
CRP(mg/L)	2.3872 ± 0.47	2.735 ± 0.78 a***	3.0855 ± 0.86 b***	3.6558 ± 1.03 c***	5.1361 ± 1.75 d***

PTH-Para Thyroid Hormone, BMI-Body Mass Index, CRP- C-reactive protein. Values are expressed as mean ± SD for the study group. a control vs mild COPD, b control vs moderate COPD, c control vs severe COPD, d control vs very severe COPD(* P < 0.05, ** P < 0.01, *** p<0.001).

5.2 TRAP staining

Many pro-inflammatory cytokines are known to increase osteoclastogenesis, since COPD provide a continuous state of systemic inflammation in the patients, differentiation of mononuclear cells stimulated with M-CSF and RANKL into osteoclasts were performed to determine the influence of the COPD at varying severity. More number of TRAP positive multinucleated cells (more than 3 nuclei) were observed in COPD subjects compared to the control. Statistical significance of $p<0.001$ between control and every severity of COPD*.

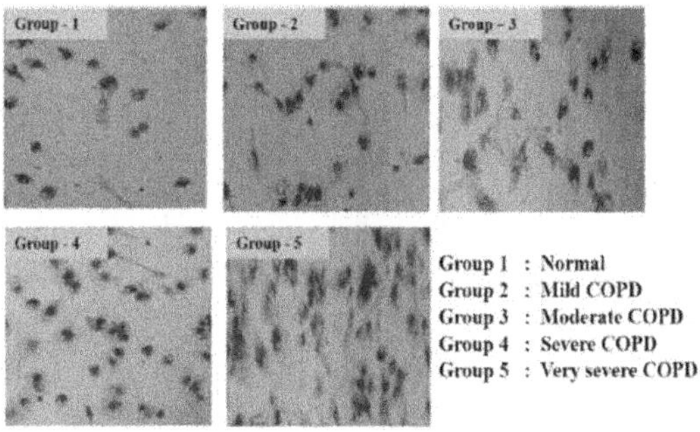

Figure 5.1. Representative images of TRAP positive osteoclast in study groups.

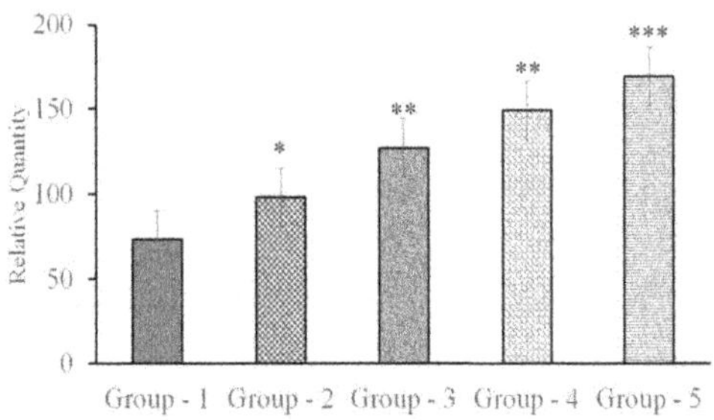

Figure 5.2. Quantitative comparison between the study groups of the numbers of TRAP positive osteoclasts.

Comparisons were made between group1 vs group2, group1 vs group3, group1 vs group4, group1 vs group5 (Group1 – control, Group2 – mild COPD, Group3 – moderate COPD, Group4 – severe COPD, Group5 – very severe COPD).

5.3 Pro-inflammatory cytokines in COPD

Pro-inflammatory cytokines were measured by ELISA. The levels of IL-1β, IL-6 and TNF-α were significantly increased in COPD subjects.

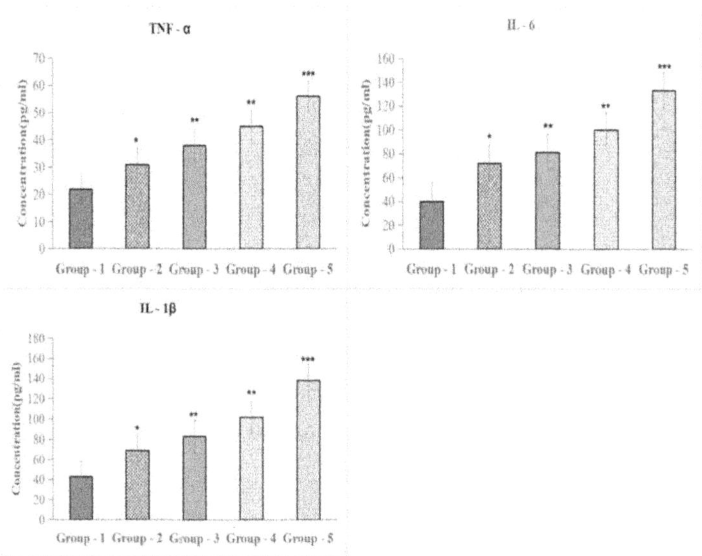

Figure 5.3 Pro-inflammatory cytokines in COPD

5.4 Expression of TRAF6, c-fos, Fra-1 and NFATc1 proteins in the study groups using immunoblot

To study the process of osteoclastogenesis in mononuclear cells obtained from the COPD patients with varying degree of disease progression, the expression of various osteoclastogenic marker proteins were analyzed after 14 day culture of the mononuclear cells under the stimulated effect of M-CSF and RANKL.

Cell lysate collected from the culture showed an increased expression of TRAF6 in mild COPD subjects which is less significant ($p<0.05$) while the expression in moderate, severe and very severe COPD subjects are highly significant ($p<0.001$) compared to the control as shown in figure 5.4.1. Severe and very severe COPD subjects showed an average of 1.5 fold increase in the TRAF6 expression compared to the control.

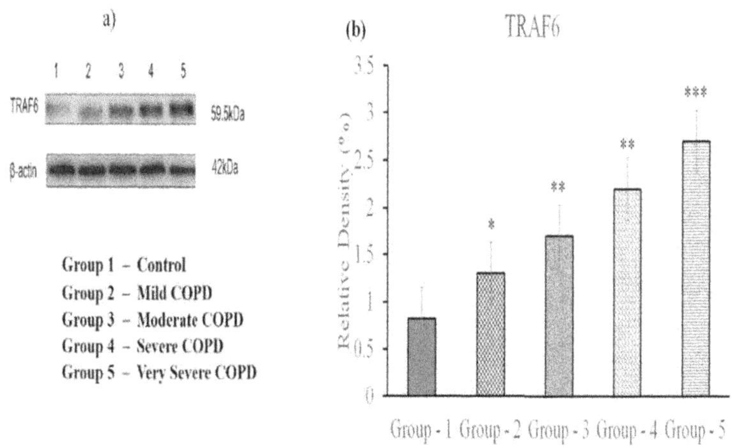

Figure 5.4.1 TRAF6 protein expression

Representative Immunoblot (a) and Quantitative comparison (b) of TRAF6 protein expression between study groups. Comparison were made between group1 vs group2, group1 vs group3, group1 vs group4, group1 vs group 5 (*$p<0.05$, **$p<0.01$, ***$p<0.001$).

Similar pattern was observed in the c-fos protein expression, mild COPD subjects showed a significance of $p<0.05$ while moderate, severe and very severe COPD subjects had a significance of $p<0.001$ compared to the healthy individuals. Figure 5.42 also reveals high variance in the c-fos expression in mild compared to other severity of the disease.

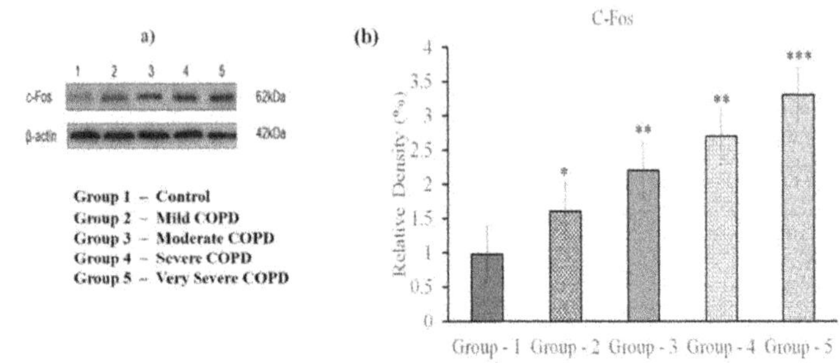

Figure 5.4.2 c-fos protein expression

Representative Immunoblot (a) and Quantitative comparison (b) of c-fos protein expression between study groups. Comparison were made between group1 vs group2, group1 vs group3, group1 vs group4, group1 vs group5 (*$p<0.05$, **$p<0.01$, ***$p<0.001$).

Fra1 displays an interesting outline of expression in the COPD patients. Mild, moderate, very severe COPD subjects exhibit a significance of $p<0.01$ whereas severe COPD subjects exhibit $p<0.001$ significance when compared to the control patients. The less significance in the very severe COPD subjects is may be due to spread of variance which is high compared to the severe, this may be due to the effect of treatment which optimizes the inflammatory condition in these patients.

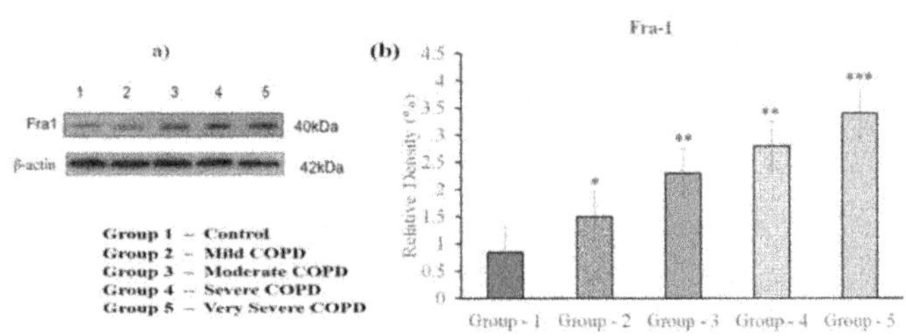

Figure 5.4.3 Fra1 protein expression

Representative Immunoblot (a) and Quantitative comparison (b) of Fra1 protein expression between study groups. Comparison were made between group1 vs group2, group1 vs group3, group1 vs group4, group1 vs group5 (*p<0.05, **p<0.01, ***p<0.001).

It is determined that the expression of the transcription factor NFATc1 in mild and moderate COPD subjects reveal a less significance of mean (p<0.01) than the severe and very severe COPD subjects (p<0.001) when compared to the normal healthy individuals (Fig.5.4.4).

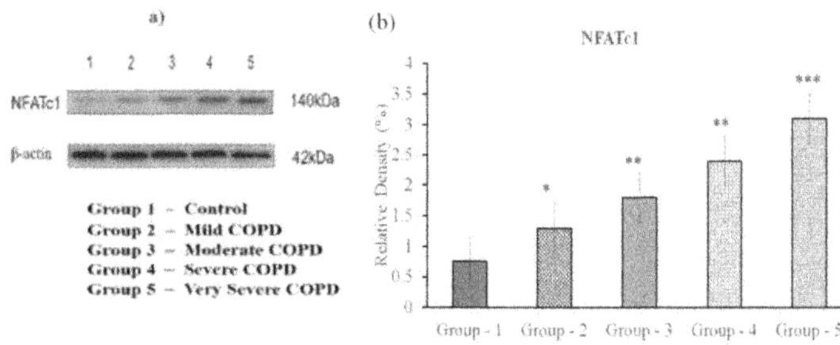

Figure 5.4.4 NFATc1 protein expression

Representative Immunoblot (a) and Quantitative comparison (b) of NFATc1 protein expression between study groups. Comparison were made between group1 vs group2, group1 vs group3, group1 vs group4, group1 vs group5 group5 (*p<0.05, **p<0.01, ***p<0.001).

5.5 Expression of osteoclast specific marker gene, CathepsinK using RT-PCR

The mRNA level of cathepsin k was assessed using RT-PCR. Mild and moderate COPD groups show a significance of mean at p< 0.01 while severe and very severe COPD groups accept the significance of mean at p<0.001 when compared to the control group (Fig.5.5).

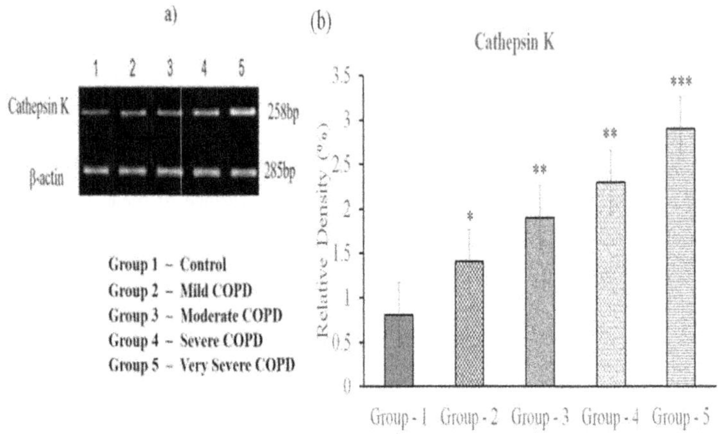

Figure 5.5. Cathepsin K gene expression.

Representative RT-PCR images (a) and Quantitative comparison (b) of Cathepsin K gene expression between the study groups. Comparison were made between group1 vs group2, group1 vs group3, group1 vs group4, group1 vs group5.

5.6. Expression levels of mitogen-activated protein kinase (MAPK) and signaling-associated proteins

MAPK signaling pathways play a crucial role in the differentiation of pre-osteoclasts cells to the mature osteoclasts. MAPK signaling pathways were examined at the protein level on osteoclasts. In severe and very severe COPD group, MAPK signaling proteins and their phosphorylated forms were highly expressed (Fig.5.6 a & b). These results indicate that COPD having osteoclastogenic and inflammatory effects.

(a)

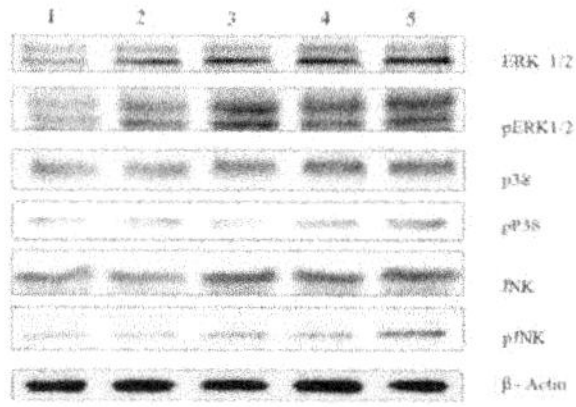

(b)

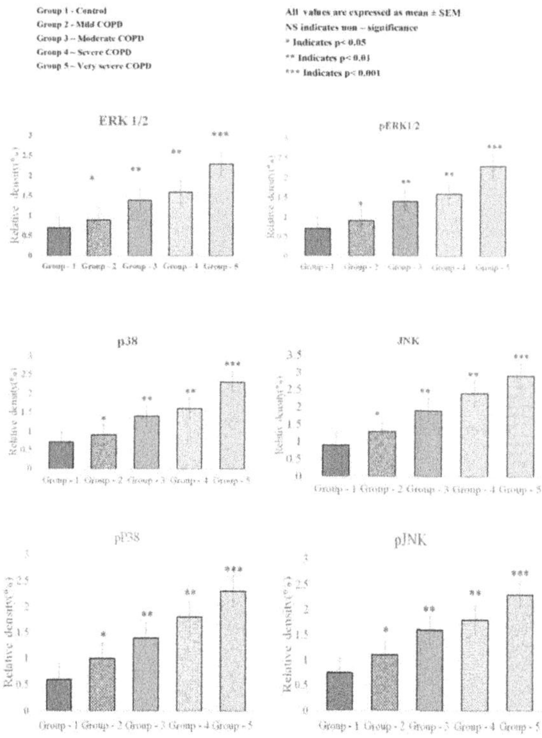

Fig.5.6 Expression levels of MAPK signaling-associated proteins in normal and COPD subjects. The expression levels of MAPK signaling-associated proteins were then analyzed by western blot analysis with corresponding antibodies. β-

actin was used as a loading and normalization control. (a) Representative blot image. (b). Relative densitometric analysis in histograms. Results were expressed as the Mean±SD. *p<0.05, **p<0.01, ***p<0.001, ns non-significance compared with control.Results represent the mean ± SD from three independent experiments.

5.7 Increased Expression of Bcl-2 and Bcl-Xl anti-apoptotic proteins

To investigate the cell death mechanism induced by COPD, the Western blot analysis of the osteoclasts of COPD patients was performed. Significant (*) changes in mild COPD group and moderate, severe and very severe showed a highly significant (***) increase in Bcl-2 and Bcl-xl respectively when compared to control (Fig.5.7)

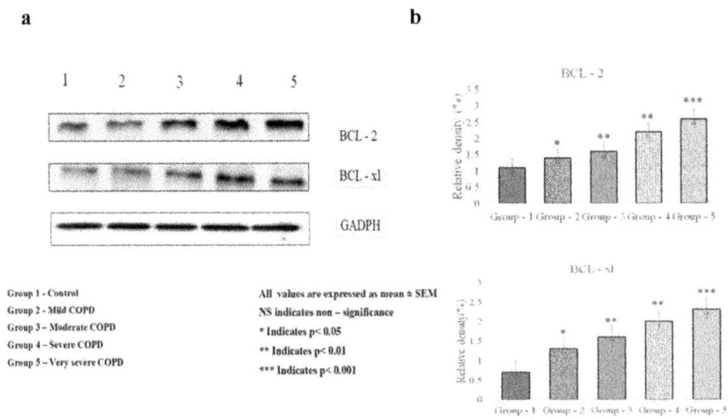

Fig.5.7 Protein expression of Bcl2 and Bclxl. (a) Representative blot image. (b). Relative densitometric analysis in histograms. *p<0.05, **p<0.01, ***p<0.001, ns non-significance compared with control. Results represent the mean ± SD from three independent experiments.

5.8. Decreased expression of pro apoptotic (Bax, Caspase-3, Caspase-9) proteins

In this, mild COPD group showed a significant decrease of Bax, caspase-3 and caspase-9. Interestingly, there is a much more significant decrease in bax, caspase 3 and caspase 9 in severe and very severe COPD groups compared with control group (Fig.5.8).

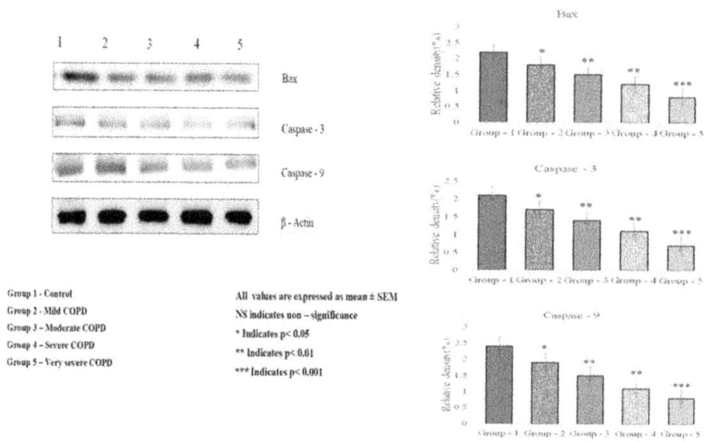

Fig.5.8 Protein expression of Bax, caspase 3 and caspase 9.

a) Representative blot image.

b) Relative densitometric analysis in histograms.

***p<0.05, **p<0.01, ***p<0.001, ns non-significance compared with control.**
Results represent the mean ± SD from three independent experiments

DISCUSSION

COPD patients are suffered from the risk of developing secondary osteoporosis due to various factors. The present study focused on to understand the expression of various osteoclastogenic markers, in order to validate the risk of increased osteoclastogenesis leading to osteoporosis and to understand the molecular mechanisms that facilitate the existence of this comorbidity in the COPD patients. The severity of COPD is also considered in this study to find the effectiveness of the different COPD conditions to support the development of the secondary osteoporosis i.e. to assess the risk of secondary osteoporosis with varying severity of COPD.

The colony stimulating factor 1 (CSF1), also known as macrophage colony-stimulating factor (M-CSF), is a secreted cytokine involves in the haematopoietic stem cells to proliferate, differentiate and be survival of monocytes, macrophages or other related cell types (Stanley *et al.,* 1997). M-CSF is a cytokine, being a smaller protein involved in cell signalling. The active site of the macromolecule is found extracellularly as a disulfide-linked homodimer, and is believed to be made by chemical change cleavage of membrane-bound precursors. M-CSF affects macrophages and monocytes in several ways, including stimulating increased phagocytic and chemotactic activity, and increased tumou r cell cytotoxicity (Nemunaitis, 1993). By interacting with its membrane receptor (CSF1R or M-CSF-R encoded by the c-fms proto-oncogene), M-CSF additionally modulates the proliferation of earlier hemopoietic progenitors and influences varied physiological processes concerned in immunology and metabolism (Fixe *et al.,* 1997). M-CSF released by osteoblasts (as a result of endocrine stimulation by parathyroid hormone) exerts paracrine effects on osteoclasts. M-CSF binds to receptors on osteoclasts inducing differentiation, and ultimately leading to increased plasma calcium levels through the resorption of bone (Han *et al.,* 2018). Supporting to the above findings, the current study also showed an increased level of calcium and parathyroid hormone in severe and very severe group of COPD (table 5.1).

Bone resorption and formation are tightly coupled in healthy individuals in a process known as bone remodeling which are mediated by three main bone cell types namely; osteocytes; osteoblasts, and osteoclasts (Raggatt *et al.*, 2010; Kini *et al.*, 2012). Abnormal osteoclastic activity leads to an impairment of bone remodeling; for example, excessive bone resorption caused by over-activation of osteoclasts is a characteristic of several bone lytic disorders. However, when there is an imbalance between formation and resorption, many bone pathologies may arise such as osteoporosis, osteopetrosis, and rheumatoid arthritis (Blair *et al.*, 2004).

Osteocytes remain embedded within the mineralized matrix of bone and are thought to translate mechanical loading into biochemical signals that affect bone remodeling (Bonewald *et al.*, 2008). Osteoblasts are responsible for the synthesis and mineralization of bone as well as modulating the differentiation of osteoclasts (Baum *et al.*, 2014). Osteoclasts are big, multinucleated cells responsible for bone resorption. They are formed by the fusion of mononuclear hematopoietic cells of the monocyte-macrophage lineage in the presence of differentiation factors, macrophage colony-stimulating factor (M-CSF) and receptor activator of nuclear factor kappa B (NF-κB) ligand (RANKL), both produced by osteoblasts (Boyce *et al.*, 2013; Teitelbaum *et al.*, 2000) .

Osteoclasts resorb bone by developing a microenvironment in which the mineral part of the bone is dissolved and the organic part is degraded (Bar-Shavit *et al.*, 2007). The osteoclast forms a sealing zone and creates a tight seal with the matrix of the bone. This sealing zone encircles the ruffled border responsible for increasing the surface area for resorption (Bar-Shavit *et al.*, 2007). To resorb bone, the generation and differentiation of osteoclasts from their precursors are crucial. The vital step in osteoclasts generation is the binding of the receptor-activator of nuclear factor κ-light chain-enhancer of activated B cells (NF-κB) ligand (RANKL) to its receptor, receptor-activator of NF-κB (RANK), in osteoclast precursors. Once RANKL binds to its receptor RANK, the downstream osteoclastogenesis signaling pathways, such as NF-κB, proto-oncogene tyrosine-protein kinase Src (c-Src), and mitogen-activated protein kinase (MAPK) pathways, including p38 MAPK, c-jun-N-terminal kinase (JNK), and extracellular signal-regulated kinase (ERK), are activated by the trimerization of tumour necrosis factor (TNF) receptor-associated factor 6 (TRAF6) (Thummuri *et al.,* 2015; Boyle *et al.,* 2003).

NF-kB is mainly activated by MAPK including extracellular signal-regulated kinase (ERK1/2), c-Jun N-terminal kinase (JNK), and p38 resulting in the expression of pro-inflammatory cytokines. Moreover, considering that lung inflammation accelerates osteoclastogenesis, the function of MAPK signaling molecules in regulating osteoclast differentiation in COPD was further studied. RANKL is over expressed by the inflammatory responses which further results in its binding to the RANK receptor on osteoclast there by causing osteoclastogenesis. The present study observed an increased level of p38, ERK1/2 and JNK in CP group (Fig.5.6 a & b). This implies that the activation of MAPK pathway might exist in COPD induced osteoclastogenesis. Increasing evidence showed that osteoclastogenesis is mainly influenced by MAPK pathway. MAPK pathway is inhibited by pharmacological inhibitors and gene silencing. This study indicates that p38, JNK and ERK signals might play a key role in intracellular signaling transduction and differentiation of osteoclasts.

Activation of NF-κB and MAPK pathways consequently leads to increased expression of transcription factors, such as proto-oncogene c-Fos (c-Fos) and the nuclear factor of activated T-cells, cytoplasmic 1 (NFATc1), which are vital for the differentiation of osteoclast precursors (Thummuri *et al.,* 2015). NFATc1 activation is a key point in the RANKL signaling cascade and known as the master regulator of osteoclast formation and function. RANKL-induced activation of c-Fos and NFATc1 is the downstream of the activation of the NF-κB and MAPK pathways (Wada *et al.,* 2006). NFATc1 increases the expression of nerve fibre cell-specific transmembrane supermolecule (DC-STAMP), that plays a vital role in bone cell formation through cell-to-cell fusion; the discharge of collagenolytic enzymes (matrix metalloproteinase nine (MMP-9), cathepsin K (CTSK), and salt resistant acid enzyme (TRAP). The

MAPKs, p-38, JNK, and ERK have all been shown to be activated once RANK is excited (Wada *et al.*, 2006;Matsumoto *et al.*, 2000; David *et al.*, 2002).

Binding of NF-κB and NFATc1 to their promoter in the nucleus controls the expression of several specific osteoclastogenesis genes, including TRAP, cathepsin K, and DC-STAMP (dendritic cell-specific transmembrane protein) (Takatsuna *et al.*, 2004; Thummuri *et al.*, 2017). The importance of the NF-κB pathway in osteoclastogenesis has been widely studied both *in vitro* and in vivo (Abu-Amer *et al.*, 2013). NF-κB deficient mice have been shown to have no osteoclasts and develop severe osteopetrosis (Xing *et al.*, 2013).

NF-κB signaling involves a group of members and a series of activation and/or inhibition steps. Under normal conditions without stimulation, the NF-κB dimer (also known as NF-κB p50/65) exists as a complex with cytoplasmic inhibitory proteins called the nuclear factor of kappa light polypeptide gene IκB family (IκBα, IκBβ, IκBε, and Bcl-3). With the stimulation of RANKL, IκB enzyme (IKK) is activated and stimulates the phosphorylation of IκB proteins at Ser32 and thirty six residues, that results in the polyubiquitination of IκB and subsequent proteasomal degradation. IκB degradation releases and activates NF-κB, which results in a translocation of NF-κB into the nucleus, which increases the transcription potential of genes involved in osteoclast differentiation (Thummuri *et al.*, 2017).

Many pro-inflammatory cytokines are known to increase osteoclastogenesis, since COPD provides a continuous state of systemic inflammation in the patients. More number of TRAP positive multinucleated cells (more than 3 nuclei) was observed in COPD subjects compared to the control (Fig. 5.1).

Multiple studies declare that the monocytes and macrophages from the PBMC that express the surface marker CD14 were the effective precursors that can be used for generations of osteoclasts (Massey and Flanagan 1999; Takeshita *et al.*, 2000). Stromal cells and osteoblasts produce two key molecules namely, M-CSF and RANKL that drives osteoclastogenesis (Teitelbaum 2000). Hence, directly adding

RANKL together with M-CSF to the cultures of osteoclast precursors could generate mature, active osteoclasts (Susa *et al.*, 2004).

The current study has revealed that the severity of COPD positively influences the process of osteoclastogenesis indicated by an increase in the number of TRAP positive multinucleated osteoclast cells in the monocyte differentiation culture of COPD subjects compared to normal as shown in Figure 5.1. The difference is significant between control group and COPD subjects of every severity group explained in the Figure 5.2. This raise in the osteoclastogenesis in the COPD groups can be owed to the presence of more pro-inflammatory monocytes in the PBMC of COPD. This is supported by the reports of Melgert *et al.*, (2003) that the higher percentage of pro-inflammatory subtypes of monocytes such as classical (CD14++, CD16+), and intermediate (CD14++, CD16+) monocytes were present in the COPD patients than the healthy individuals but this strongly depends on age.

In the present study, COPD has been identified as an important modulator of inflammation and osteoclast differentiation. It is hypothesized that IL-1β, IL-6 and TNF-α play a key role in activating osteoclasts that terminate in net bone resorption. In the present study, IL-1β, IL-6 and TNF-α were increased in COPD, severe and very severe group suggesting an inflammatory response during the progression of the disease (Fig. 5.4.1a). There were consistent results in different studies demonstrating the increased levels of pro-inflammatory cytokines in very severe COPD group.

A separate study by Aldonyte *et al.*, (2003) reveals that the LPS-stimulated secretion of specific pro-inflammatory molecules such as IL-6 and MCP-1 from circulating monocytes differs between healthy and COPD subjects. Excessive reports suggests that the inflammatory cytokines such as IL-1, IL-6, and TNF-α produced by the monocytes directly induce osteoclastogenesis and thereby increase bone resorption (Hardy and Cooper 2009; Zupan *et al.*, 2013).

Tumor necrosis factor (TNF) Receptor-Associated Factor 6 (TRAF6) could be a member of TRAF super molecule family, that plays a important role in each innate and adaptive immune responses by mediating signal transduction from members of the cytokine taxonomic group, the toll-like receptor/interleukin-1 receptor (TLR/IL-1R) family, and also the TCR (Inoue, Gohda, & Akiyama, 2007; Kobayashi, Walsh, & Choi, 2004).

To study the process of osteoclastogenesis in mononuclear cells obtained from the COPD patients with varying degree of disease progression, the expression of various osteoclastogenic marker proteins were analyzed after 14 day culture of the mononuclear cells under the stimulated effect of M-CSF and RANKL. Cell lysate collected from the culture showed an increased expression of TRAF6 in mild COPD subjects which was less significant ($p<0.05$) while the expression in moderate, severe and very severe COPD subjects was highly significant ($p<0.001$) compared to the control as shown in figure 5.3. Severe and very severe COPD subjects showed an average of 1.5 fold increase in the TRAF6 expression compared to the control.

TRAF6 also plays an important role in osteoclastogenesis by transducing the receptor mediated signals to cytoplasmic downstream targets. RANK does not have intrinsic kinase activity and it depends on the TRAF family of proteins for further transmission of signal through kinase activity particularly, TRAF6 (Armstrong *et al.*, 2002; Galibert *et al.*, 1998; Wong *et al.*, 1998). Various other receptors, such as CD40, TLR4, and those recognizing IL-1 and IL-17 also bind TRAF6, but unlike RANK, they are not uniquely capable of promoting osteoclast differentiation (Rong *et al.*, 2007; Wu and Arron 2003).

This may be either due to unambiguous number of TRAF6-binding sites in RANK or presence of unique adaptor proteins that are not associated with other TRAF6- binding receptors (Cao *et al.*, 1996; Kadono *et al.*, 2005). Studies showed that TRAF6-deficient mice developed severe osteopetrosis due to impaired osteoclastogenesis (Kobayashi *et al.*, 2003; Lomaga *et al.*, 1999). In addition, TRAF6-deficient osteoclast precursors obtained from spleen fail to differentiate into mature osteoclasts *in vitro* even in the presence of both M-CSF and TRANCE. AP-1 is a collection of related transcription factors belonging to the Fos (c-Fos, FosB) and

Jun (c-Jun, JunB, JunD) families which dimerize in various combinations through their leucine zipper region. Fos/Jun form heterodimers with high affinity and are the predominant form of AP-1 in most cells, whereas Jun/Jun homodimers bind with low affinity and are less abundant (Manning & Davis, 2003). AP-1 may be activated by various cytokines, including TNF-α and IL-1β, via several types of protein tyrosine kinase (PTK) and mitogen-activated protein (MAP) kinases, in particular, Jun-N-terminal kinase (JNK), which themselves activate a cascade of intracellular kinases (Saklatvala, 2004). AP-1, like NF-κB, regulates many of the inflammatory and immune genes that are overexpressed in asthma. Indeed, many of these genes require the simultaneous activation of both transcription factors that work together cooperatively. Interestingly, AP-1 has recently been shown to be involved in glucocorticoid receptor DNA accessibility by regulating chromatin structure (Biddie *et al.*, 2011). There is evidence for increased expression of c-Fos in bronchial epithelial cells in asthmatic airways (Demoly *et al.*, 1992) and an even greater expression in patients with severe, treatment-insensitive asthma (Adcock & Lane, 2003; Loke *et al.*, 2006), and many of the stimuli relevant to asthma that activate NF-κB that will also activate AP-1.

RANK activates the transcription factor complex AP-1 partly through an induction of its critical component, c-fos (Takayanagi *et al.*, 2002; Wagner 2005). It can also be suggested that c-fos is crucial for AP-1 interaction with its specific transcriptional partner that is required in osteoclastogenesis (H. H.Kim *et al.*, 2003). c-fos is an important mediator of osteoclastogenesis, and mice lacking c-fos developed osteopetrosis caused by a differentiation defect in the osteoclast lineage (Ikeda *et al.*, 2004), complete block of osteoclast differentiation (Grigoriadis *et al.*, 1994; Wang *et al.*, 1992) and because of a lack of osteoclasts.

c-Fos is a proto-oncogene and a part of a bigger Fos family of transcription factors which includes c-Fos, FosB, Fra-1 and Fra-2 (Milde *et al.*, 2005). It has been mapped to chromosome region 14q21→q31. c-Fos encodes a 62 kDa protein, which forms heterodimer with c-jun (part of Jun family of transcription factors), resulting in the formation of AP-1 (Activator Protein-1) complex which binds DNA at AP-1 specific sites at the promoter and enhancer regions of target genes and converts extracellular signals into changes of gene expression (Chiu *et al.,* 1988).

The present study examined the ability of COPD of varying severity to induce Fra-1 and c-fos expression *in vitro,* of the study groups. Figure 5.4.2 depicts that the c-fos expression is increased in the osteoclast culture of COPD groups relatively compared to control group. In addition, the up-regulation of c-fos expression resulted in a concomitant increase in the expression of Fra-1 in COPD groups compared to control as shown in Figure 5.5. This is consistent with the study of Vaz *et al.,* (2015), who reported that cigarette smoke, a major determinant of COPD, strongly stimulates Fra-1 expression in lung epithelial cells. Interestingly, in a separate study, it was observed that an elevated level of Fra-1 expression in the lungs of cigarette smoke-exposed mice have developed emphysema which is a form of COPD. Fra-1, which is a transcriptional target of c-fos during osteoclast differentiation, also rescues the differentiation blockade of c-fos deficient osteoclast precursor cell both *in vivo* and *in vitro* (Matsuo *et al.,* 2000). Recent data using retroviral gene transfer into c-fos mutant osteoclast precursors *in vitro* have also shown that fra-1 can efficiently complement for the absence of c-fos (Matsuo *et al.,* 2000). Importantly, the total restoration of osteoclast differentiation was achieved in knock in mice generated by the insertion of the Fra-1 gene into the c-fos locus (Fleischmann *et al.,* 2000). But Fra-1 deficient mice do not exhibit osteopetrosis (Eferl *et al.,* 2004). This suggests that Fra-1 has an ability to compensate for the loss of c-fos but is not the exclusive downstream molecule of c-fos. Moreover, the osteoclast differentiation factor RANKL (Karsenty and Wagner 2002) induces Fra-1 transcription in a c-fos dependent manner, thereby establishing a link between RANK signaling and the expression of AP1 proteins during osteoclast differentiation (Matsuo *et al.,* 2000). These studies that were performed in cell culture and animal models provide compelling preliminary evidence that AP-1 signaling plays a role in COPD and osteoclastogenesis.

Similar pattern was observed in the c-fos protein expression, mild COPD subjects showed a significance of $p<0.05$ while moderate, severe and very severe COPD subjects had a significance of $p<0.001$ compared to the healthy individuals. Figure 5.4 also reveals a high variance in the c-fos expression in mild compared to other severity of the disease.

Fra1 displayed an interesting outline of expression in the COPD patients. Mild, moderate, very severe COPD subjects exhibited a significance of $p<0.01$ whereas severe COPD subjects exhibit $p<0.001$ significance when compared to the control patients. The less significance in the very severe COPD subjects may be due to spread of variance which is high compared to the severe; this may also be due to the effect of treatment which optimizes the inflammatory condition in these patients.

Nuclear factor of activated T-cells (NFAT) is a family of transcription factors shown to be important in immune response. One or more members of the NFAT family are expressed in most cells of the immune system. NFAT is also involved in the development of cardiac, skeletal muscle, and nervous systems. NFAT was first discovered as an activator for the transcription of interleukin-2 in T cells, as a regulator for T cell immune response, but has been found to play an important role in regulating many other body systems (Pan *et al.*, 2013).

The NFAT transcription factor family consists of five members NFATc1, NFATc2, NFATc3, NFATc4, and NFATc5 (Crabtree *et al.*,2002). NFATc1 through NFATc4 are regulated by calcium signaling, and are known as the classical members of the NFAT family. Calcium signal is important to NFAT activation as a result of calmodulin (CaM), a widely known metallic element sensing element supermolecule, activates the serine/threonine enzyme calcineurin (CN). Activated CN dephosphorylates the serine-rich region (SRR) and SP-repeats within the amino termini of NFAT proteins, leading to a conformational amendment that exposes a nuclear localization signal, leading to NFAT nuclear import. NFATc1 is expressed in peripheral lymphoid tissue (Rao *et al.*,1997). NFAT also plays a role in rheumatoid arthritis (RA), an autoimmune disease that has a strong pro-inflammatory component.

TNF-α, a pro-inflammatory cytokine, activates the calcineurin-NFAT pathway in macrophages (Pan *et al.,* 2013).

In the present study, the expression of the transcription factor NFATc1 in mild and moderate COPD subjects revealed a less significance of mean ($p<0.01$) than the severe and very severe COPD subjects ($p<0.001$) when compared to the normal healthy individuals. Figure 5.4.4 indicates an increased expression of NFATc1 in COPD subjects and the increase is proportional to the severity of the disease compared to the healthy subjects. The induction of NFATc1 is a hallmark event in the cell fate determination of osteoclasts. In a genome-wide search for the RANKL-inducible genes specifically required for the terminal differentiation of osteoclasts, NFATc1 was shown to be strongly induced by RANKL (Asagiri *et al.,* 2005; Takayanagi *et al.,* 2002). The mRNA of NFATc1 is induced selectively and potently by RANKL (Asagiri *et al.,* 2005; Takayanagi *et al.,* 2002). Extensive evidences support the explanation that the NFATc1 expression is dependent on the TRAF6, NF-κB and c-fos pathways which are activated by RANKL, suggesting an integral role of NFATc1 in RANKL signaling. The *in vitro* observation of NFATc1−/− embryonic stem cells shows inhibition of osteoclast differentiation and the finding that ectopic expression of NFATc1 causes bone marrow-derived precursor cells to undergo osteoclast differentiation in the absence of RANKL (Takayanagi *et al.,* 2002). Since NFATc1 induction was shown to be impaired in TRAF6−/− cells (Takayanagi *et al.,* 2002), it has been suggested that NFATc1 is one of the key target genes of NF-κB in the early phase of osteoclastogenesis.

Liu *et al,* reported the significant increased expression of NFATc 1 in the rat muscle fibers in response to moderate-intensity exercise. These findings suggest that the increase in calcium/calmodulin-dependent phosphatase (CaN) activity induced by moderate physical exertion leads to upregulation, and possibly activation, of NFATc1. CaN is an important regulator of muscle growth and development. It is involved in regulating the maturation of myocytes and differentiation of muscle fibers in adults. However, the role of NFAT isoforms in muscle development and physiology has been rarely studied. Altogether, these findings have identified a molecular mechanism that an increase in $Ca2^{+}$ concentration in the muscle in turn bind to the calmodulin–calcineurin enzyme complex, and modulate the activity of NFAT proteins. Phosphorylation and subsequent translocation of NFATs from the cytosol to the nucleus is tightly regulated by calcineurin. Nuclear NFATs bind to corresponding nucleotide recognition sequences and induce transcription of the target genes (Rao *et al.,* 1997). Several studies have elucidated the diversity of the NFAT family of transcription factors, and their functional association with other transcription factors to regulate the expression of inducible genes. Studies showed that NFATs play an important role in skeletal muscle physiology, by mediating a selective response to slow muscle-specific motor neuron activity. *In vitro* experiments demonstrated that fast to slow myosin conversion of skeletal muscle cells can be induced by a ten-fold increase in intracellular calcium concentration (Kubis *et al.,* 1997). This finding further supports the present results on the increase in the concentration of calcium in severity of the disease.

The mRNA level of cathepsin k was assessed using RT-PCR. Mild and moderate COPD groups showed a significance of mean at $p< 0.01$ while severe and very severe COPD groups showed the significance of mean at $p<0.001$ when compared to the control group. mRNA analysis of cathepsin K indicated in figure 5.5, revealed that the expression is governed by the inflammatory condition showing an increased expression in COPD subjects with respect to the severity of the disease compared to the control subjects. Cathepsin K is activated in an acidic bone microenvironment to efficiently degrade type I collagen, the most abundant extracellular protein in bone matrix (Inaoka *et al.,* 1995). Cathepsin K is preferentially and highly expressed in the osteoclasts from all species that have been studied (Inaoka *et al.,* 1995; Tezuka *et al.,* 1994; Yamaza *et al.,* 1998). This is now known to be true as cathepsin K knockout mice exhibit a phenotype of osteopetrosis (Gowen *et al.,* 1999; Saftig *et al.,* 1998).

Cathepsin K, a member of the cathepsin family of lysosomal cysteine proteinase, plays a critical role in bone resorption which is regulated by NFATc1. Cathepsin K was found to be secreted by lung epithelial cells, which possesses both collagenase and elastase activities, capable of degrading fibrillar collagen at several sites, contrary to MMPs that cleave collagen at one specific site (Buhling *et al.,* 2004). The expression of cathepsinK was detected mainly in the alveolar macrophages of the smoke-exposed animals (Mercer *et al.,* 2004). Although the role of cat K is well known in lung fibrosis, very little is known about its potential role in COPD. Only one study has demonstrated an increased expression of cathepsin K in lung homogenates of COPD patients (Golovatch *et al.,* 2009). In addition, they showed that chronic smoke exposure significantly increased cat K expression by alveolar macrophages. Golovatch et al reported the elevated expression of cathepsin K in the human lung extracts of patients with emphysema confirming the clinical relevance of cathepsinK in human disease. The increased activity of such potent proteolytic enzyme is likely responsible for the development of emphysema in the guinea pig lung (Golovatch *et al.,* 2009). Furthermore, osteoclastic bone resorption was inhibited by cathepsin K antisense oligodeoxynucleotide *in vitro* (Inui *et al.,* 1997). Therefore, this finding is noteworthy for its contribution to the understanding of the pathogenesis of COPD suggesting the dysregulated activity of cathepsin K.

Recently, an increasing number of data suggests an important mechanism involved in the development of COPD; the apoptosis of structural cells in the lung might possibly be an important upstream event in the pathogenesis of COPD. There is an increase in apoptotic alveolar epithelial and endothelial cells in the lungs of COPD patients. Since this is not counterbalanced by an increase in proliferation of these structural cells, the net result is destruction of lung tissue and the development of emphysema.

Apoptosis is a key mechanism allowing multicellular animals to tightly regulate the cell growth (Baetu and Hiscott 2002). Necrosis, "accidental" cell death, is a pathological process which occurs when cells are exposed to a serious physical or chemical insult. During necrosis, the loss of membrane integrity leads to the influx of water and extracellular ions. Intracellular organelles, most notably the mitochondria and the entire cell swell and rupture and the cytoplasmic contents are released into the extracellular fluid. During apoptosis, the coordinated morphological and biochemical changes occur within the nucleus, cytoplasm, organelles, and plasma membrane (Cohen 1993).

Apoptosis can be triggered through two major pathways, one implicating death receptor ligation and the other the release of cytochrome c from mitochondria (Baetu and Hiscott 2002). The death receptor pathway is initiated by the ligation of members of the tumour necrosis factor (TNF) family, such as TNF-α and Fas-ligand, to their respective ligands, TNF receptor 1, and Fas (Baetu and Hiscott 2002). These "death-inducing" receptors recruit the death-inducing signaling complex through interaction with adaptor proteins such as Fas associated death domain protein (FADD). In turn, FADD recruits caspase-8. Caspase-8 activation leads to either direct activation of caspase-3, or to cleaving of Bid, a member of the bcl-2 family, which in turn targets mitochondria for cytochrome c release (Baetu and Hiscott 2002).

The mitochondrial pathway can be triggered by both external and internal stimuli. Members of the bcl-2 family of proteins, like bcl-2, bax, and bad, gather at the surface of mitochondria, where they compete to regulate cytochrome c release, which leads to caspase-9 activation. Bcl-2 is an antiapoptotic and bad and bax are proapoptotic members of this family (Baetu and Hiscott 2002). Akt is a serine-threonine kinase that phospholylates and thereby inactivates the proapoptotic proteins bad and caspase 9 and elevates the expression of the antiapoptotic protein bcl-2 (Datta et al 1999). Both pathways converge at the level of caspase-3 activation. Caspases are proteolytic enzymes, the executioners of apoptosis.

The osteoclast undergoes spontaneous apoptosis through the activation of the death receptor pathway or mitochondrial apoptosis pathway (Kroemer *et al.*, 2007). The intrinsic mitochondrial apoptotic pathway is characterized by the release of cytochrome c from permeabilised mitochondria into cytosol and activation of caspases. This release is mediated by activated Bax and deregulation of Bcl-2.

These activated proteins, triggers mitochondrial outer membrane permeabilisation (MOMP), which thereby releases cytochrome c and activates caspase 9, which in turn activates caspase 3 and 7 which leads to apoptotic cell death (Kroemer *et al.*, 2007). Research into the molecular mechanisms of the apoptotic stimulus has uncovered the Bcl-2 protein family that is thought to function as apoptosis regulators (Ma *et al.*, 2009). Bcl-2 family members are capable of forming homo and heterodimers with one another suggesting that the overall ratio of pro to anti apoptotic regulators may determine whether a cell is condemned to die of apoptosis or not (Li *et al.*, 2013).

The osteoclast undergoes spontaneous apoptosis through the activation of the death receptor pathway or mitochondrial apoptotic pathway (Kroemer *et al.*, 2007). Interestingly, osteoclasts derived from COPD groups had significantly reduced expressions of pro-apoptotic markers like Bax and Caspases (Fig.5.8) whereas increased expressions of anti-apoptotic markers like Bcl-2 and Bcl-xl (Fig.5.7).

Increased caspase 3 and 9 expressions were found by western blot suggesting that the increased pro-apoptotic function of caspase 3 and 9 might play an important role in the pathogenesis of COPD leading to osteoporosis (Fig. 5.8). Also, the detection of increased caspase 3 and caspase 9 activities is an evidence of apoptotic mechanisms are lapsed in progress.

Therefore, it is assumed that COPD decreased the permeability of the mitochondrial membrane and suppressed the release of cytochrome C and other pro-apoptotic factors into the cytoplasm, thereby inhibiting the caspase-dependent apoptosis of osteoclasts.

CONCLUSION

The present study reports that development of osteoporosis is promoted by the enhanced expression of osteoclastogenic markers and their expression depends upon the disease severity. COPD could also induce the increased expression of signaling pathways which promote this heightened osteoclastogenesis and thus promoting secondary osteoporosis. This molecular study opens a new area of research and drug development that could improve the quality of life in COPD subjects

SUMMARY

The present study focuses principally on the elevated development of osteoclasts based on the severity of COPD patients ranging from mild to severe disease. This study deciphers the intricate intracellular signaling pathways responsible for the development of increased osteoclastogenesis. Further this study has also explored the altered osteoclastogenic markers and their involvement in the development of osteoporosis.

This study has revealed that increasing severity from mild, moderate and severe, there was an elevated expression of osteoclastogenic molecules like NFATc1, c-fos, Fra-1, cathepsin K and TRAF-6. This reveals that increase in the osteoclasts are directly associated with the disease severity.

In addition, this study explores the signaling pathways which could contribute to the osteoclast development in COPD patients. MAP kinase and NF-κB pathways are critical pathways that could increase osteoclastogenic markers and this study reports that these signaling cascades are highly expressed and they could attribute to this COPD-dependent secondary osteoporosis.

9 781805 250661

Printed by BoD™in Norderstedt, Germany